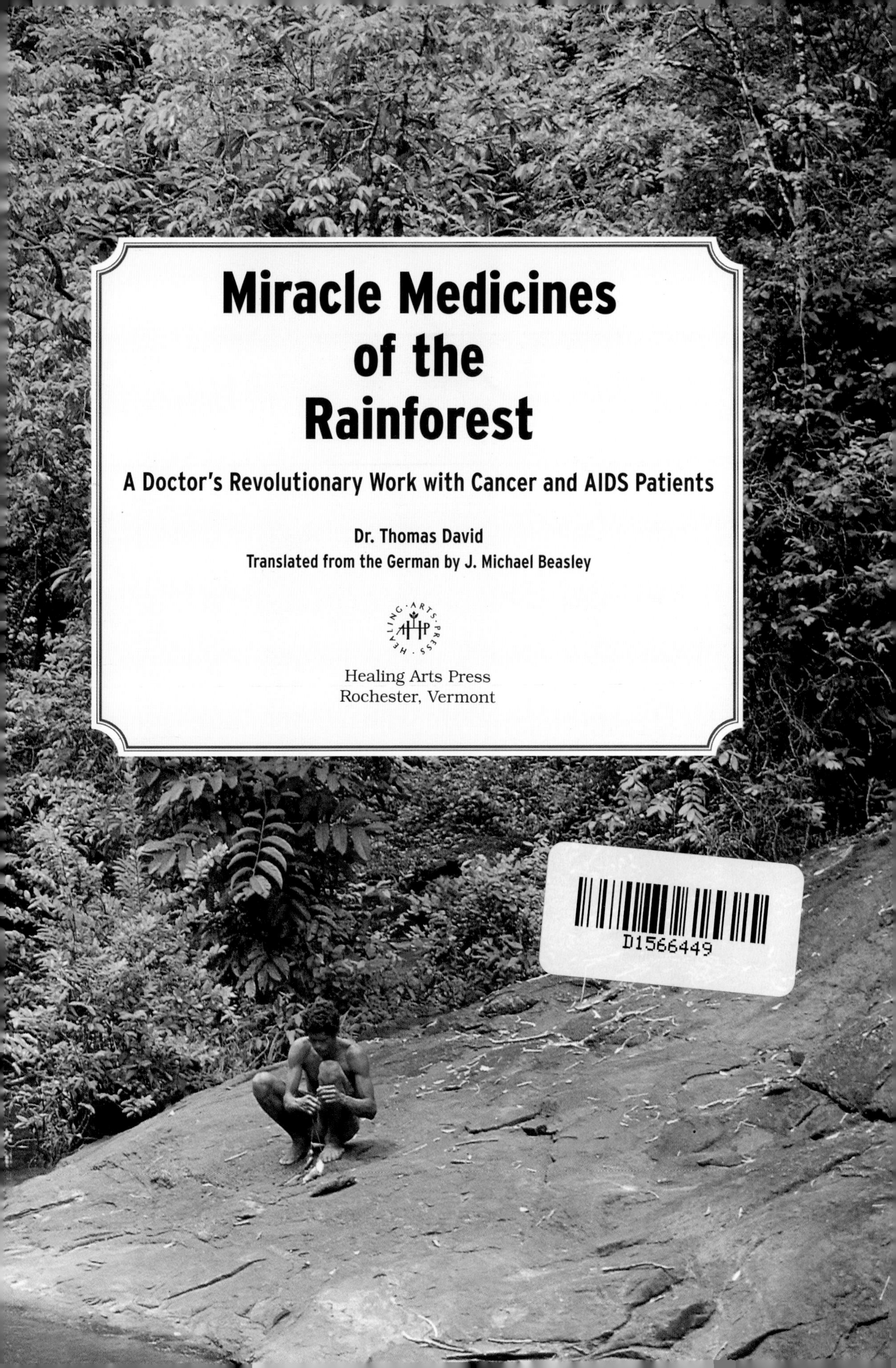

Miracle Medicines of the Rainforest

A Doctor's Revolutionary Work with Cancer and AIDS Patients

Dr. Thomas David

Translated from the German by J. Michael Beasley

HEALING ARTS PRESS

Healing Arts Press
Rochester, Vermont

Healing Arts Press
One Park Street
Rochester, Vermont 05767
www.gotoit.com

First U.S. edition published by Healing Arts Press 1997

Originally published in German under the title *Medizin der Schamanen* 1996

General editor: Werner Stanzl

Note to the reader: This book is intended as an informational guide. The remedies, approaches, and techniques described herein are meant to supplement, and not to be a substitute for, professional medical care or treatment. They should not be used to treat a serious ailment without prior consultation with a qualified health-care professional.

Library of Congress Cataloging-in-Publication Data
David, Thomas.
[Medizin der Schamanen. English]
Miracle medicines of the rainforest : a doctor's revolutionary work with cancer and AIDS patients / Thomas David. — 1st U.S. ed.
p. cm.
ISBN 0-89281-746-1 (alk. paper)
1. Herbs—Therapeutic use. 2. Cancer—Alternative treatment. 3. AIDS (Disease)—Alternative treament. 4. Medicinal plants—Brazil. 5. Materia medica, Vegetable—Brazil. 6. Rain forest plants—Brazil. 7. Herbal teas. 8. Immunological adjuvants. I. Title.
RM666.H33D3713 1997 97-22873
615'.32'0981—dc21 CIP

Printed and bound in Italy

10 9 8 7 6 5 4 3 2 1

Text design and layout by Kristin Camp
This book was typeset in Bookman

Healing Arts Press is a division of Inner Traditions International

Distributed to the book trade in Canada by Publishers Group West (PGW), Toronto, Ontario

Distributed to the health food trade in Canada by Alive Books, Toronto and Vancouver

Distributed to the book trade in the United Kingdom by Deep Books, London

Distributed to the book trade in Australia by Millennium Books, Newtown, N.S.W.

Distributed to the book trade in New Zealand by Tandem Press, Auckland

Distributed to the book trade in South Africa by Alternative Books, Ferndale

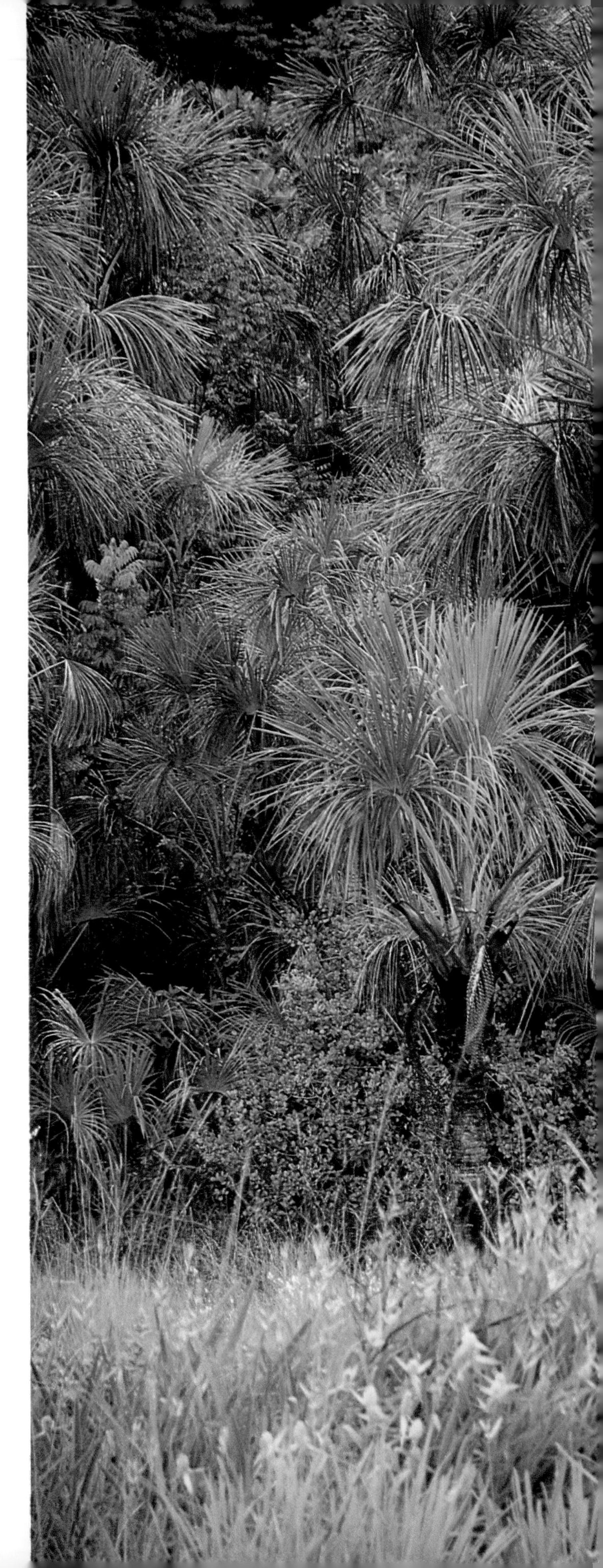

Miracle Medicines of the Rainforest

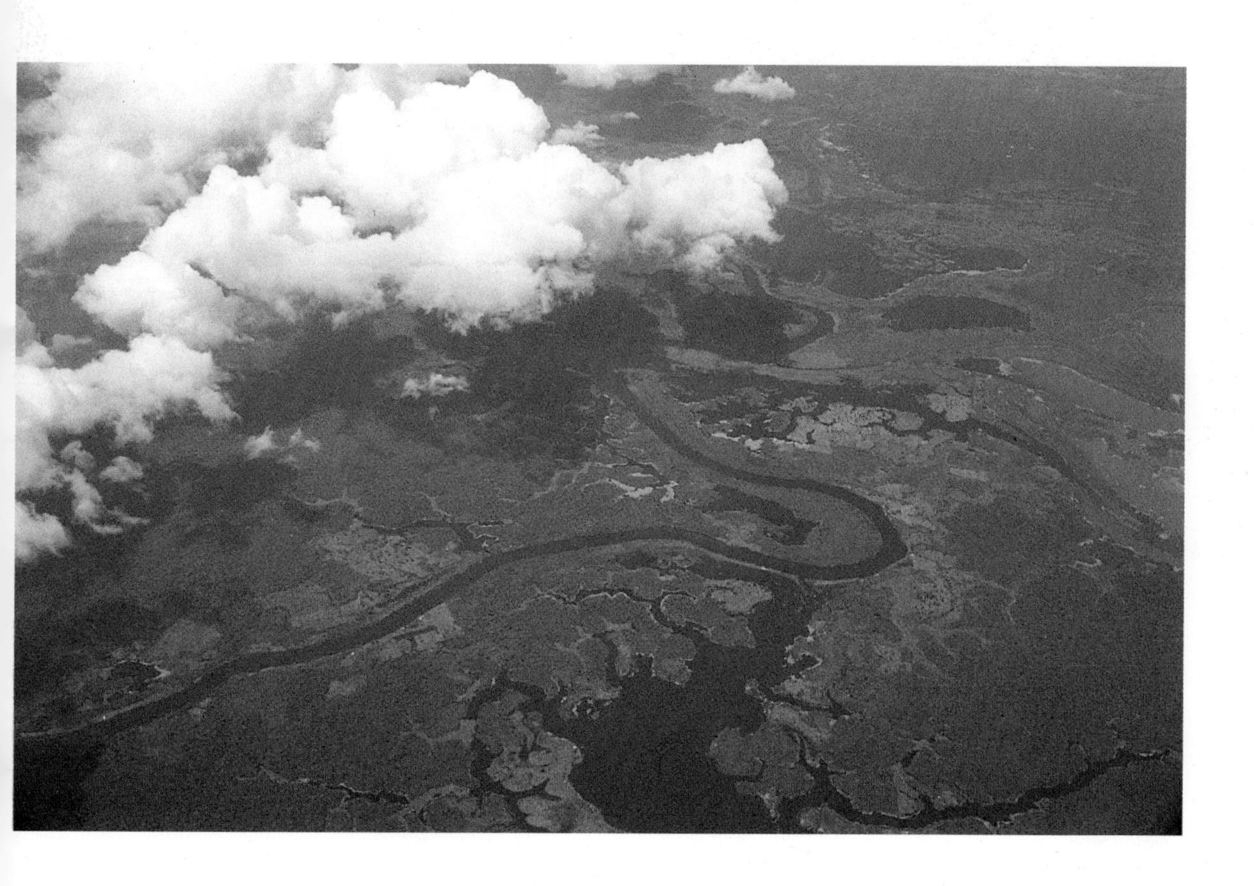

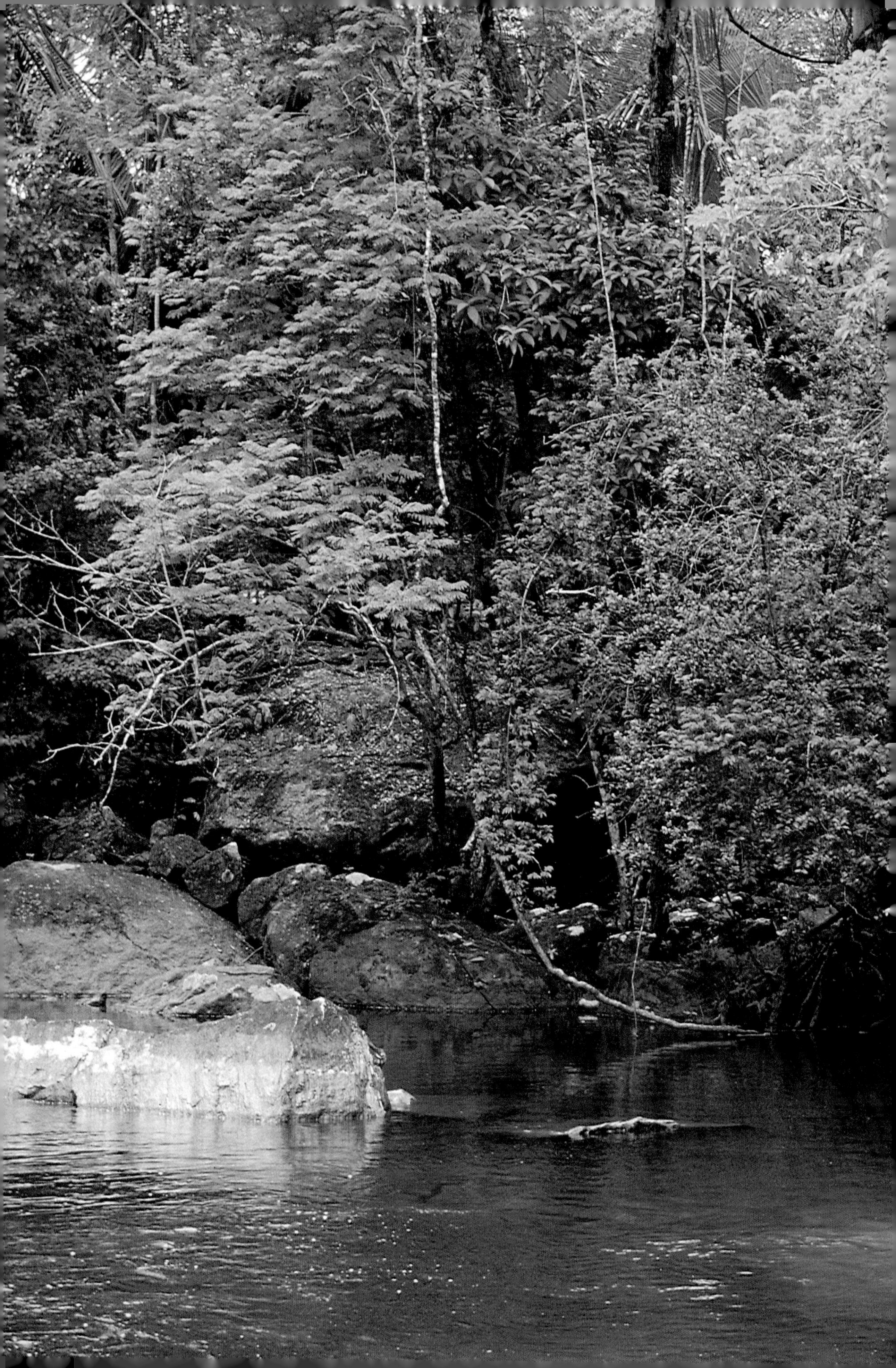

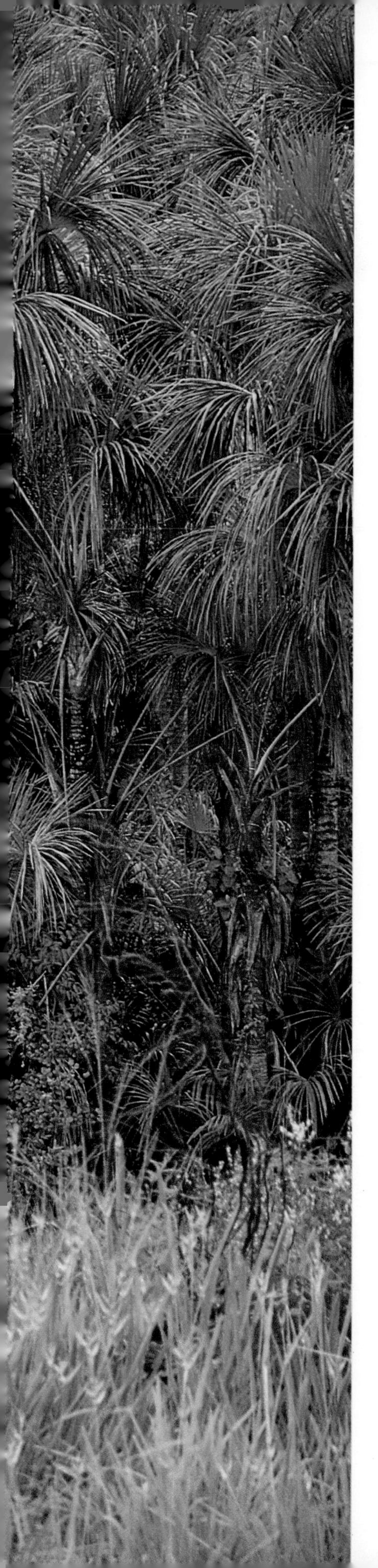

Contents

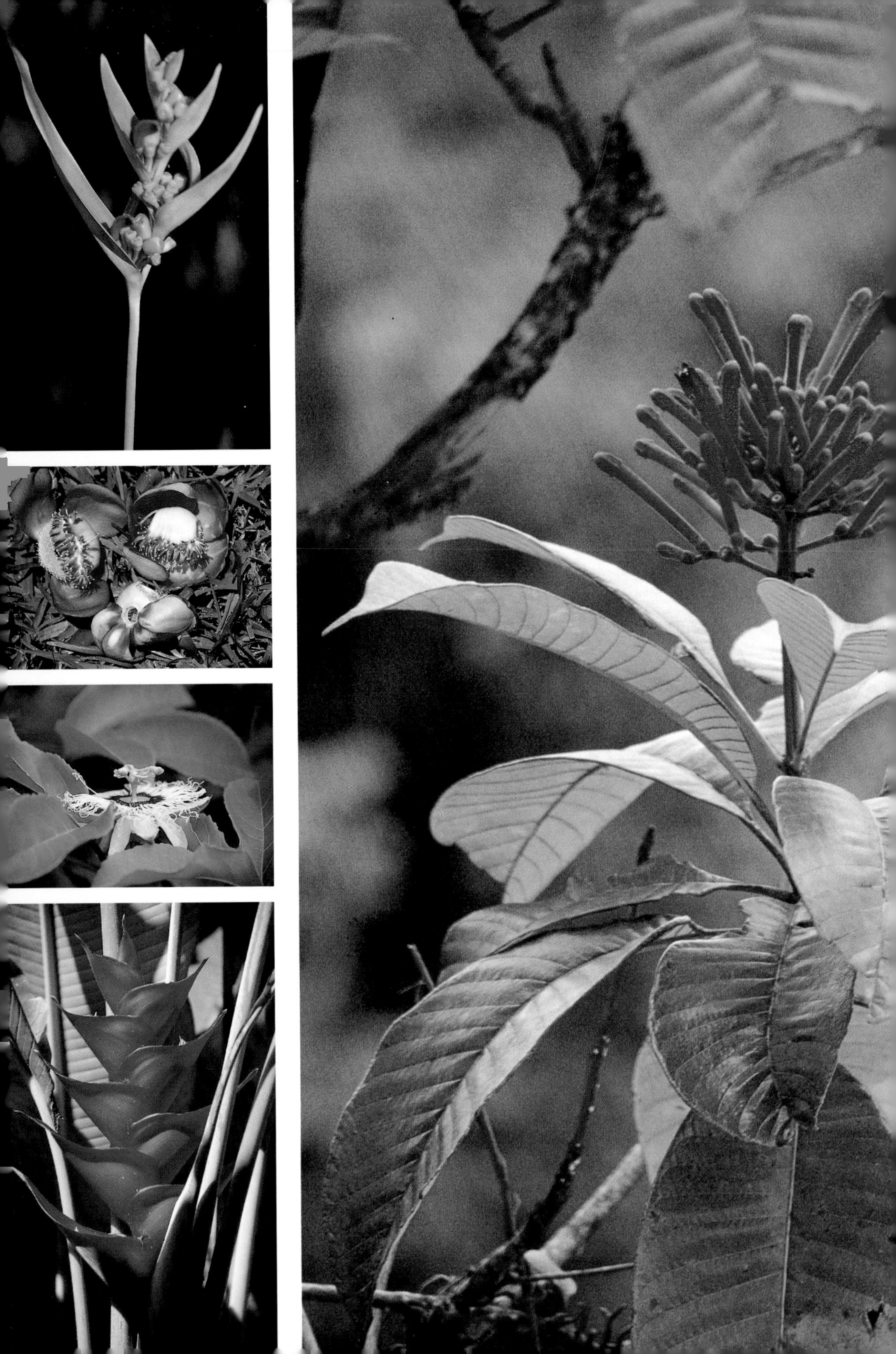

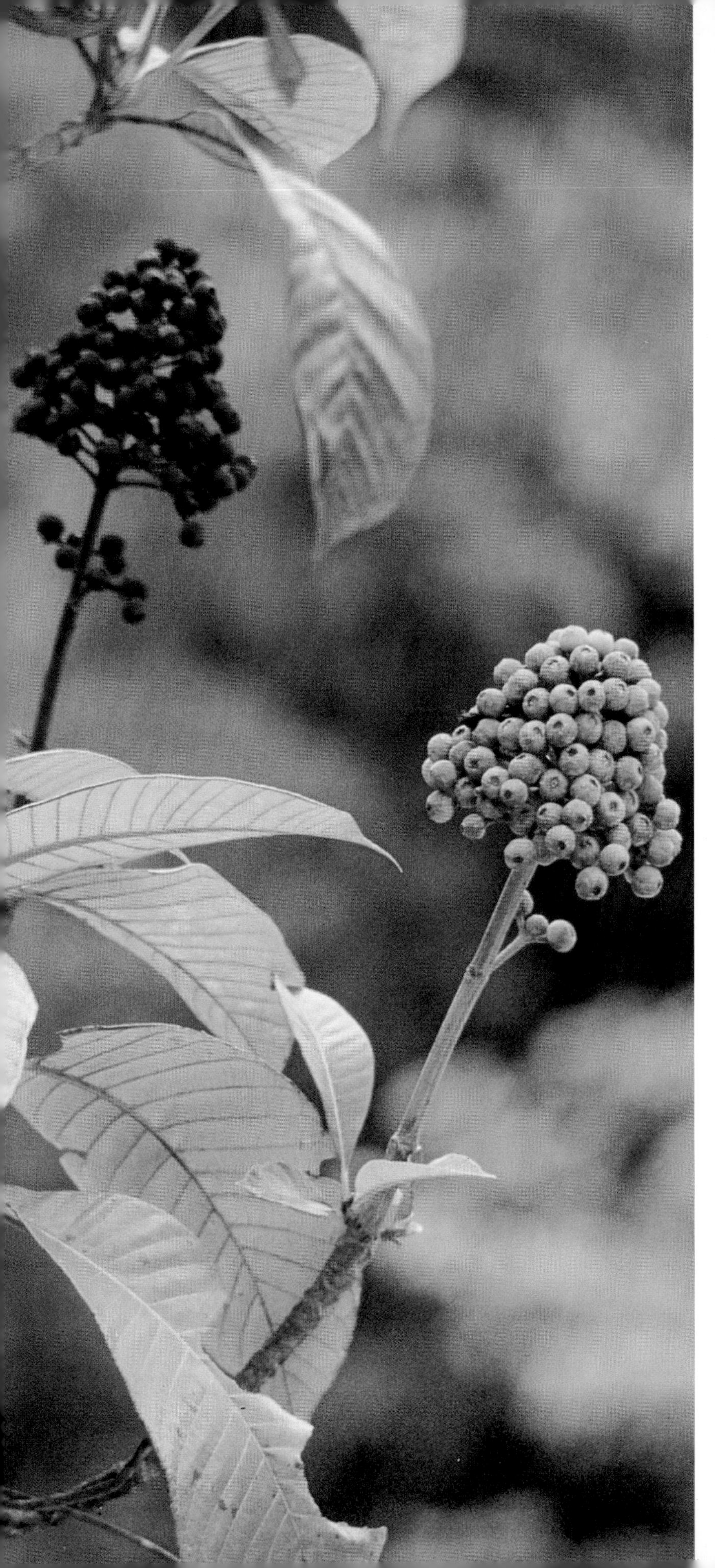

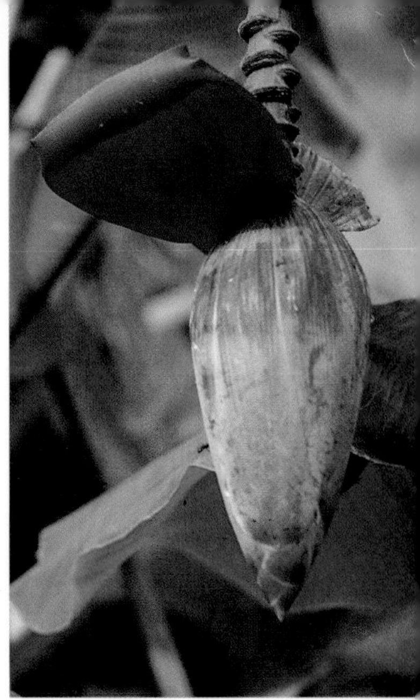

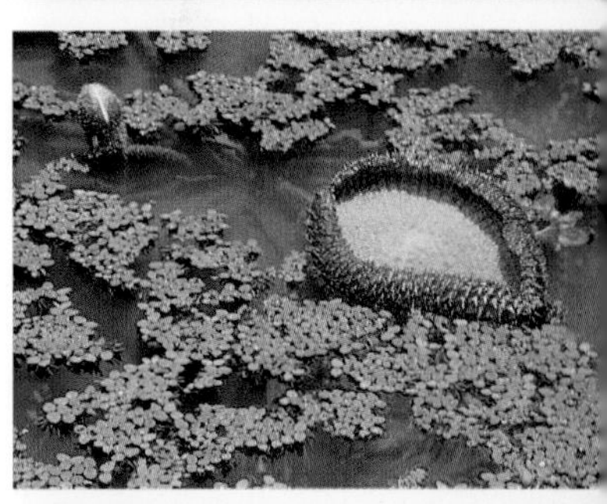

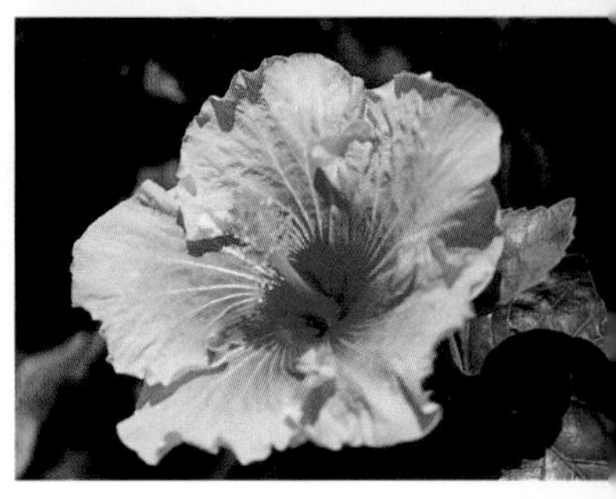

The variety of flora and fauna in the rainforest is astounding. In an area of just a few square kilometers there can be found more varieties of plants than are found in all of Europe. In sixty million years of evolution these species have learned how to survive in a hostile environment.

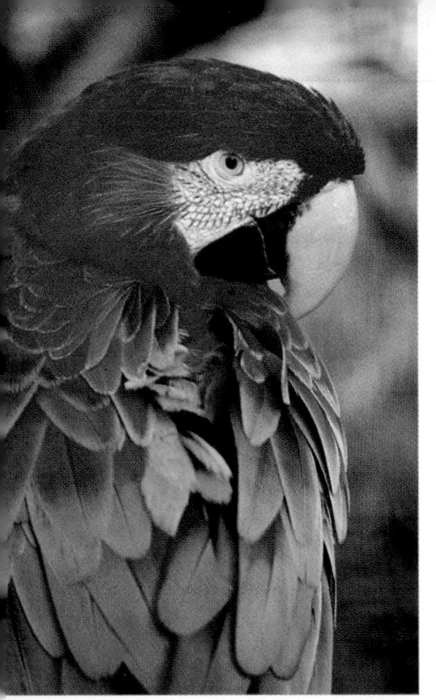

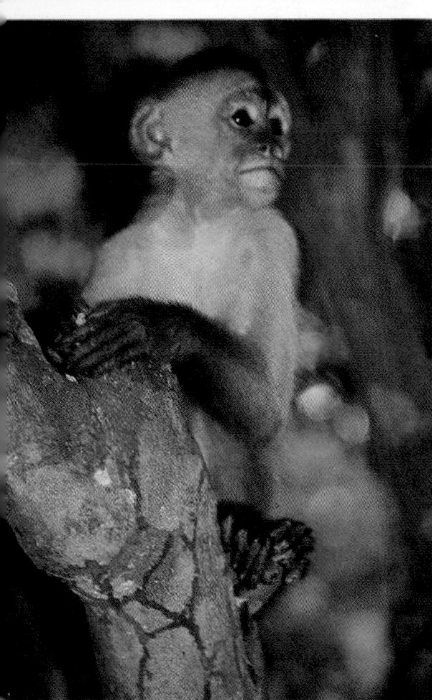

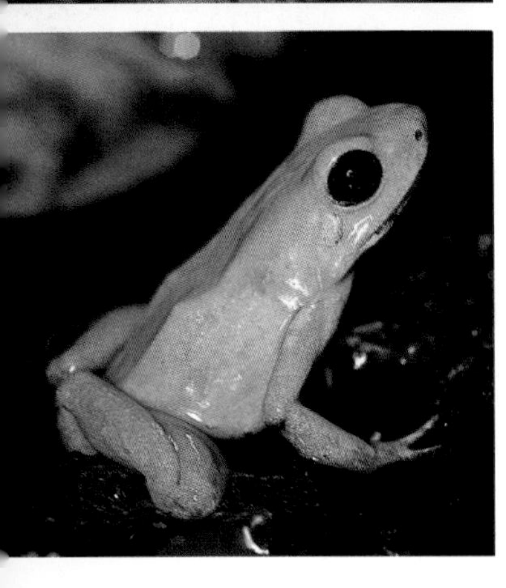

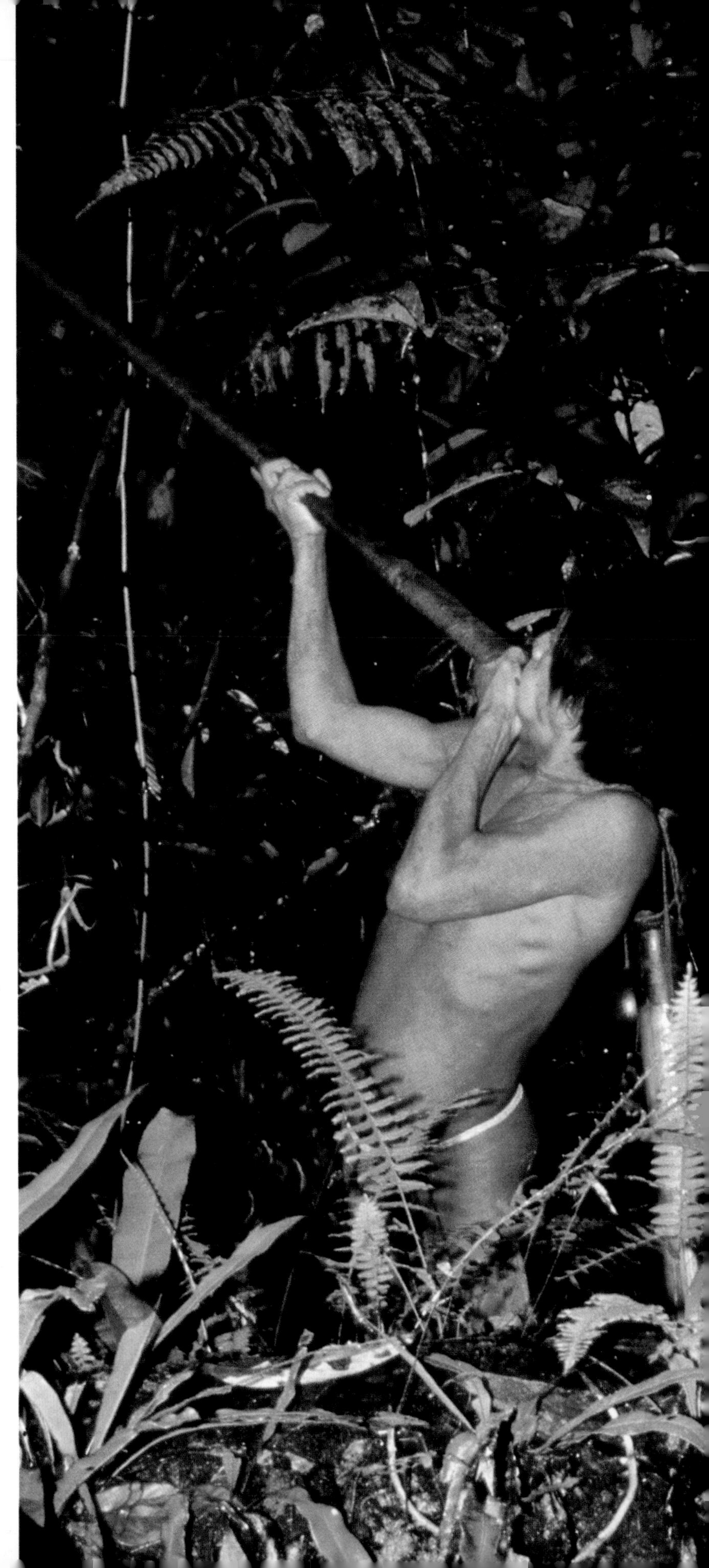

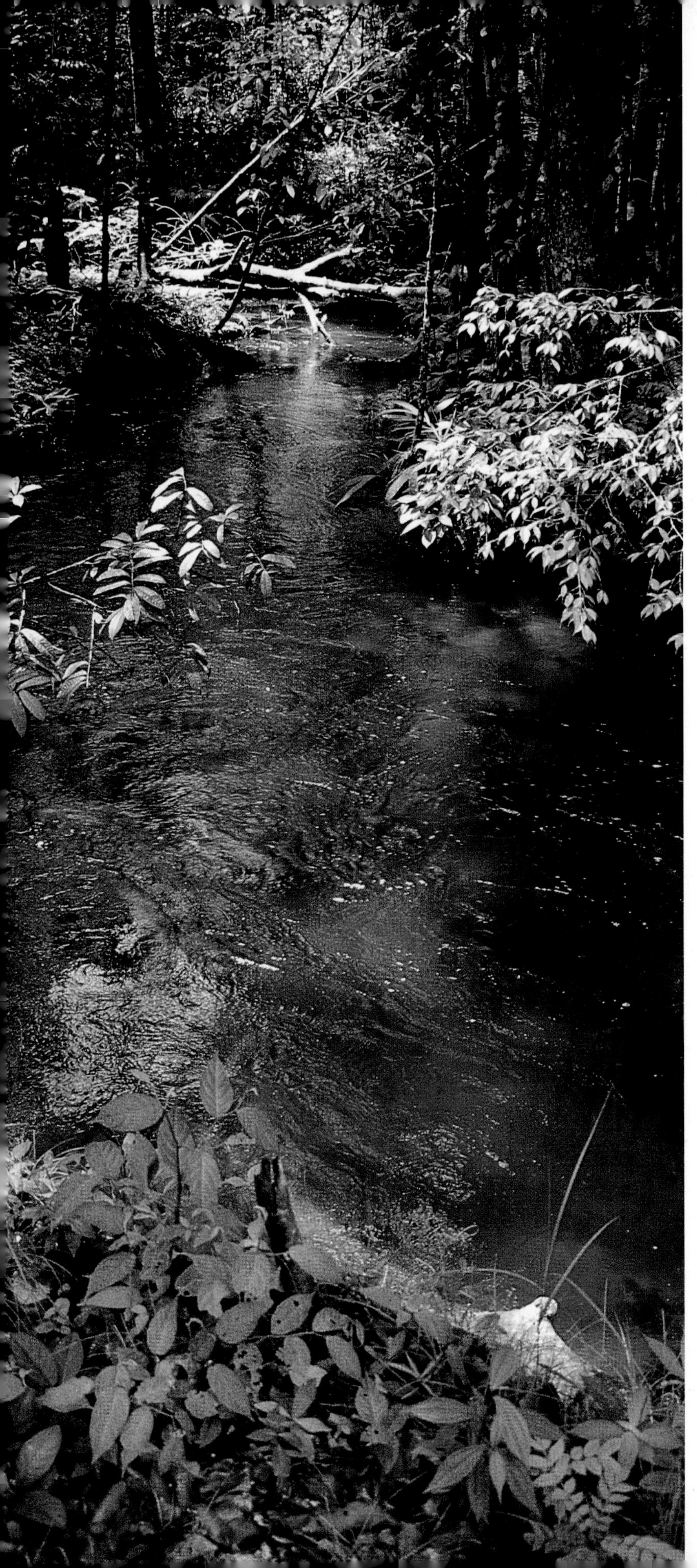

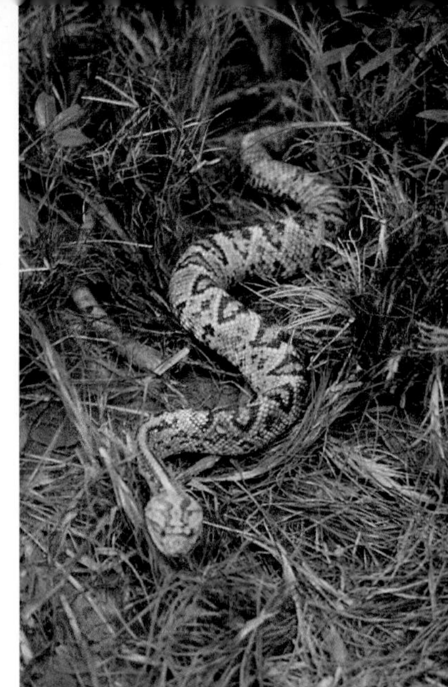

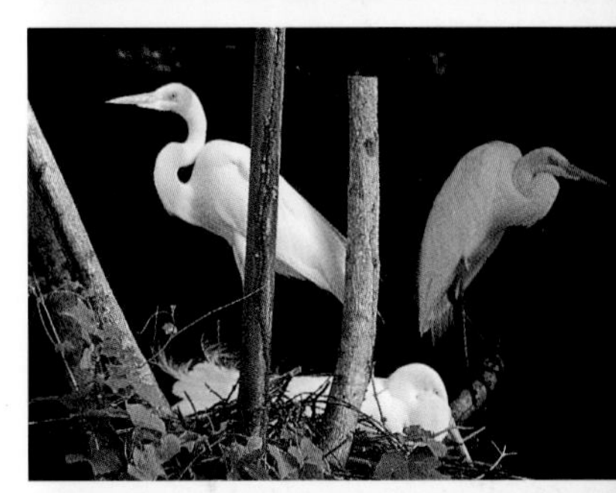

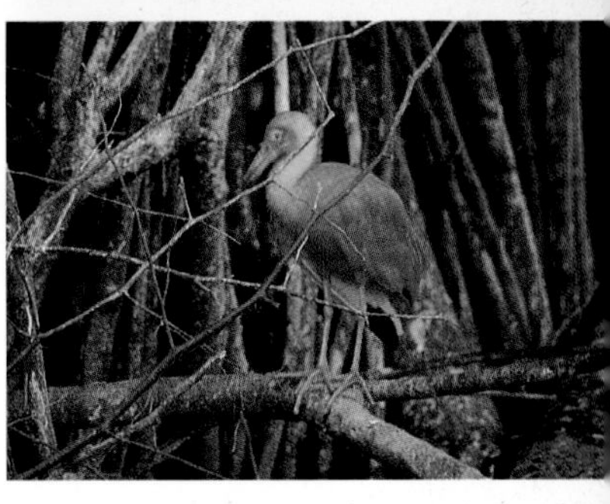

Parrots, monkeys, poisonous frogs, snakes, and water birds: the rainforest is a storehouse of the world's most valuable treasures. It contains billions of combinations of genetic information. Despite vocal protests, the rainforest is still being put to the torch every day.

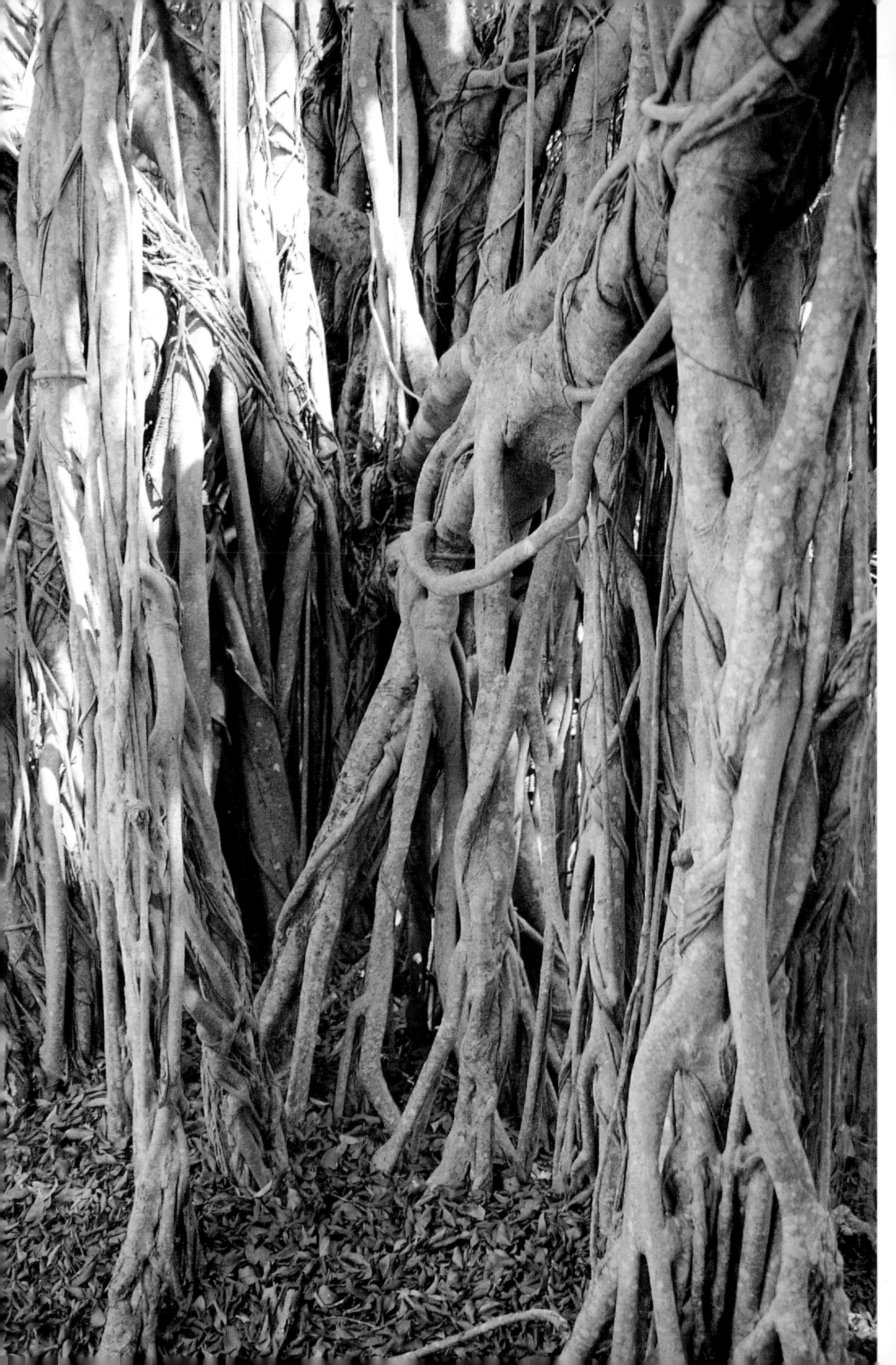

Foreword

Opposite: The above-ground roots function like gills during a flood. They extract oxygen from the water, allowing the tree to survive.

Perhaps I'm an incurable optimist, but I believe that humanity will soon stop burning the rainforest. I attribute this comforting notion to an urgent television news report in January 1996: "La Fenice, the venerable opera house in the City of Canals, the stage of many world premieres of Verdi, has burned down." My TV screen was filled with pillars of black smoke coming from the former cultural mecca, and firefighters fought the fight of their lives to save what was left of the aging and weak structure. The next morning, further reports came in: "Donors from around the world have contributed millions of deutschemarks to help restore La Fenice to its former glory. The opera house should reopen in 1998."

These reports confirmed my belief that humanity is prepared to make sacrifices in order to save and maintain what is important. For this reason, I cannot imagine that people will stand by helplessly and watch as priceless treasures are burnt down for short-term profits. These treasures are hidden in the equatorial rainforest. The rainforest does not just serve to regulate the world climate; it is above all a library with an irreplaceable collection. In it are stored untold billions of bits of information on the structure, metabolism, growth, and survival mechanisms of flora and fauna. If these plants or animals should become extinct, this information will be lost forever. Only here, and nowhere else, can they be observed and studied. Until now we have understood at best only a small part of this treasure. The researcher of the rainforest is faced with a situation similar to that of a researcher of the cosmos: we know that there are billions of suns and planets out there, but unimaginable distances separate us from them.

Forty years ago a trip across the Atlantic was as daunting as a round trip to the moon would be today. When compared to the sixty million years that the rainforest has existed, this forty years seems like only a minute. In this minute, however, its existence has been devastated more by the hands of humans than by all the climatic changes, volcanic eruptions, and meteorite showers throughout the past sixty million years. More recently, since the

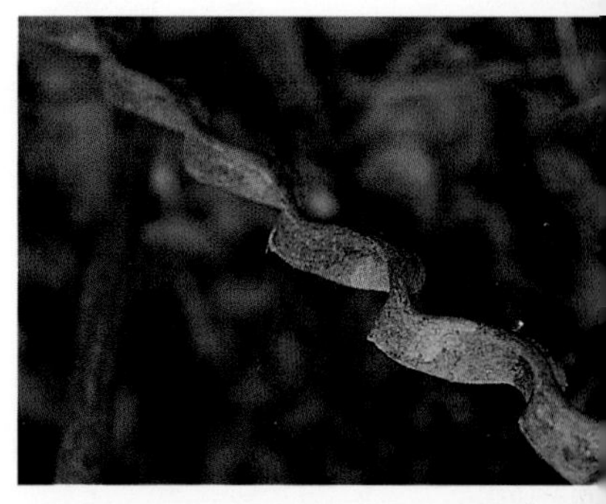

Vines can grow up to one hundred meters long. This "turtle ladder" looks like the work of a master metalsmith.

The thorn tree knows, after sixty million years of evolution, that only birds can guarantee its survival. Birds eat seeds in the fruit, which are later passed out undigested. The thorny bark prevents animals from climbing the tree, but birds can land uninjured and then carry the seeds and fruit in all directions.

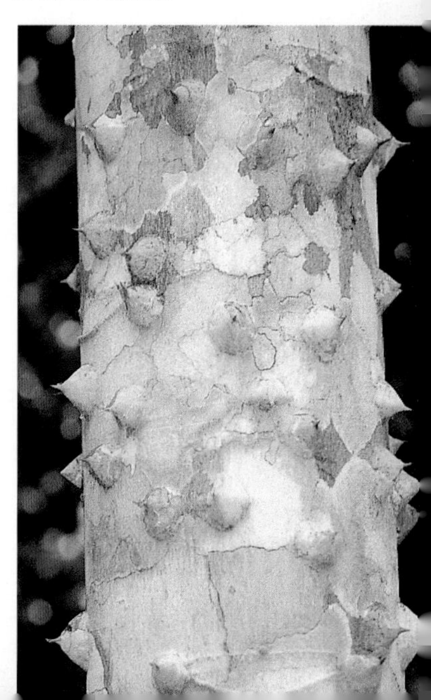

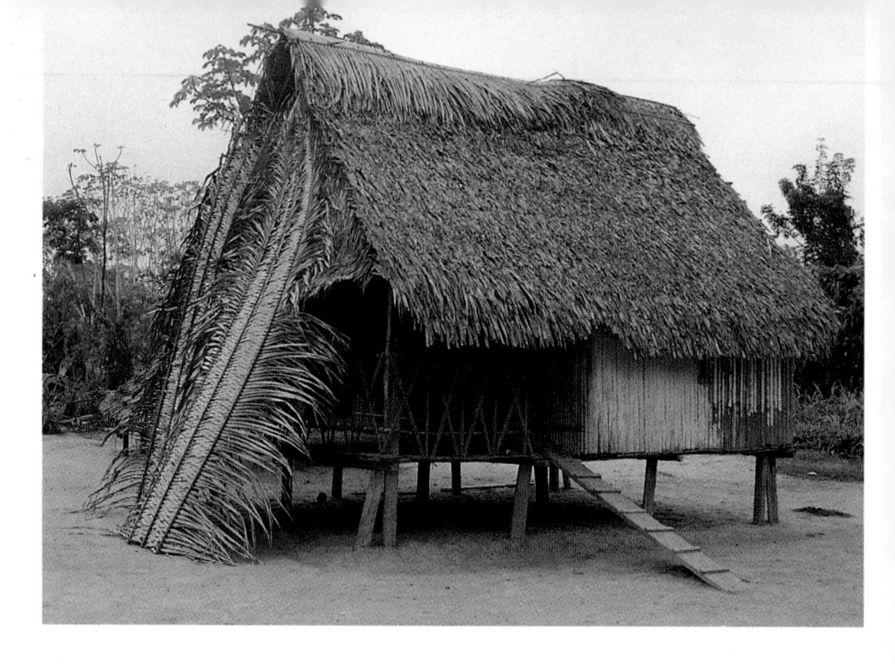

A single-family house in an Indian village on the Rio Ucayali. These types of villages are found wherever Indian existence has been threatened from road construction, burning of forests, or gold mining.

When Indians move to a village or city, the women seem to adapt more readily than the men, who are for the most part unwilling to do anything except the hunting and fighting.

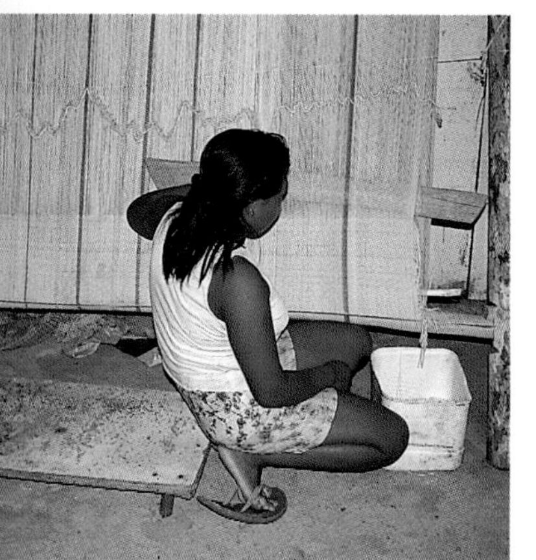

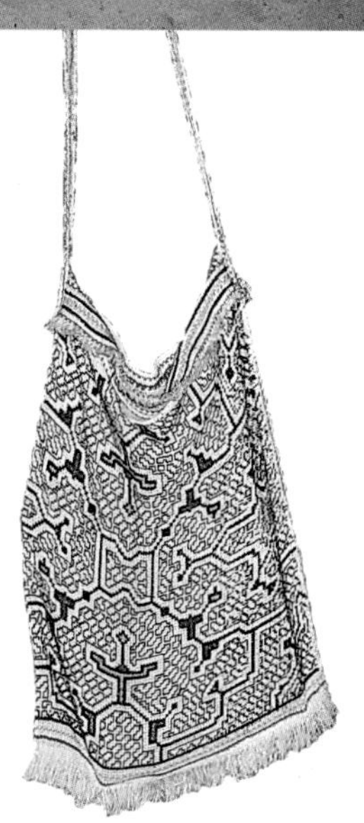

discovery of quinine, we have come to think of the rainforest as our own "green pharmacy." This natural medication for malaria and other tropical illnesses comes from the dried bark of the South American cinchona tree.

Another plant extract made headlines in 1963. Shamans in Madagascar had taught researchers the wonders of an evergreen with pink blossoms. Years of clinical research showed that this plant contains an agent which is highly effective against leukemia. Thanks to its effectiveness, today four out of five children can survive an illness which has been previously absolutely fatal. And who could have predicted more than twenty years ago that at the dawn of the new millennium Western surgeons would be using a deadly poison used by the Amazon Indians? Anyone who made such a claim would have received pitying smiles from friends and colleagues, or would have been sized up for a straitjacket. Today, however, the *Brockhaus Encyclopedia* defines "curare" as "a deadly poison, an alkaloid mixture, which the indigenous tribes of South America derive from the bark of *Strychnos toxifera*. Curare paralyzes the nerves which control the movements of muscles and it is used as an anesthetic during surgery."

By a happy coincidence, I had the chance to come into contact with shamans and medicine men of the rainforest Indians. They have shown me plants which, when used in the right mixtures and in conjunction with a specified diet, can lengthen the life expectancy and improve the quality of life of "incurable" cancer patients.

Modern medicine is in the very early stages of developing an awareness of the powers of Nature and its uses in medicine. But if our natural treasures are destroyed, this awareness may never fully develop.

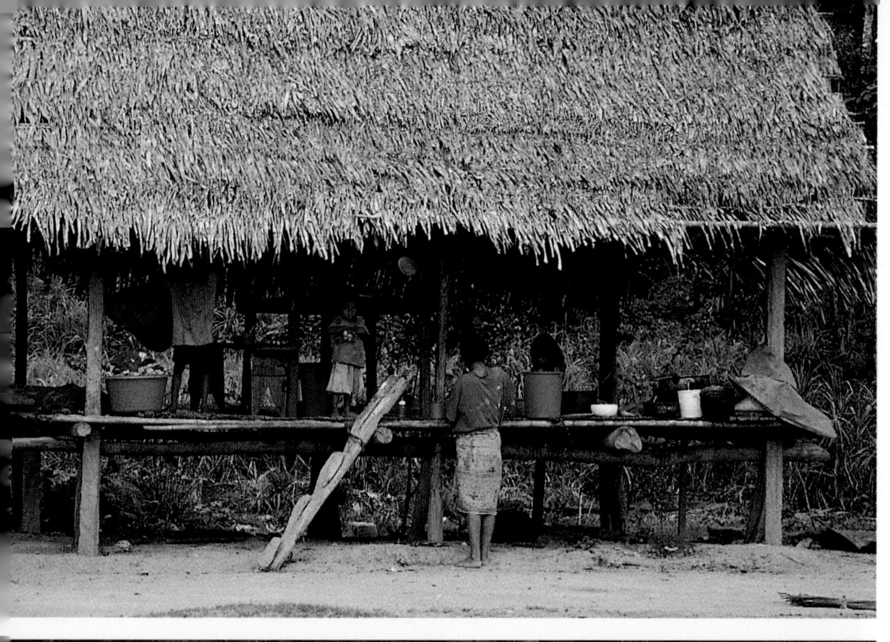

Left: The materials are modest, but Indian pile huts are masterpieces. Air circulates freely under the roof, and the floor functions as a surface for eating and working. If there is an especially high flood, they build an "upper deck."

Center: Living room, workroom, and bedroom all in one—all with the strong smells of the forest.

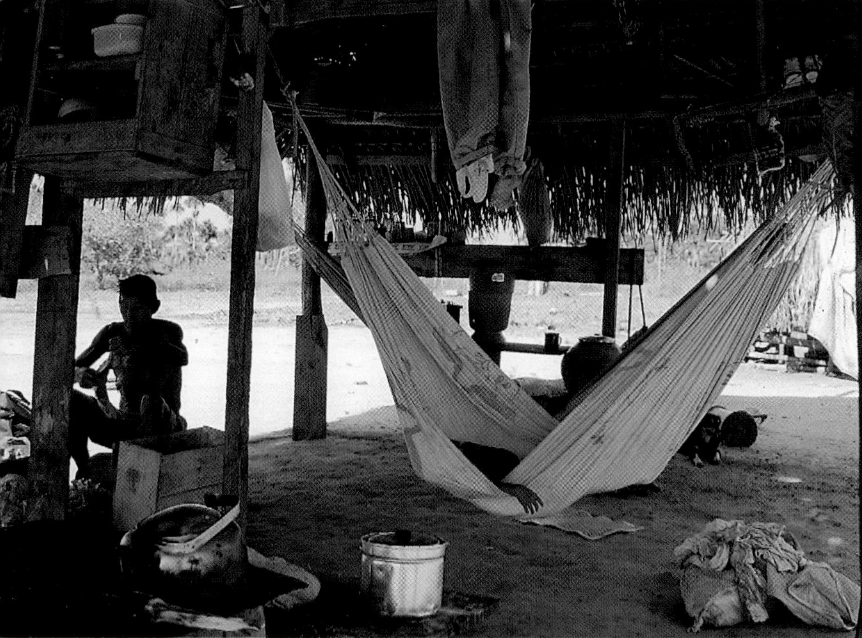

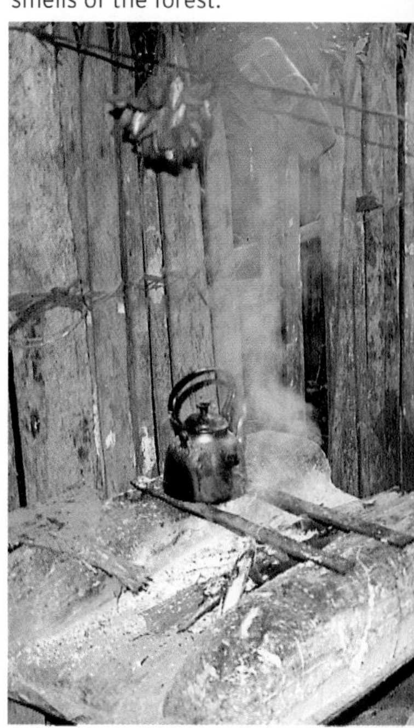

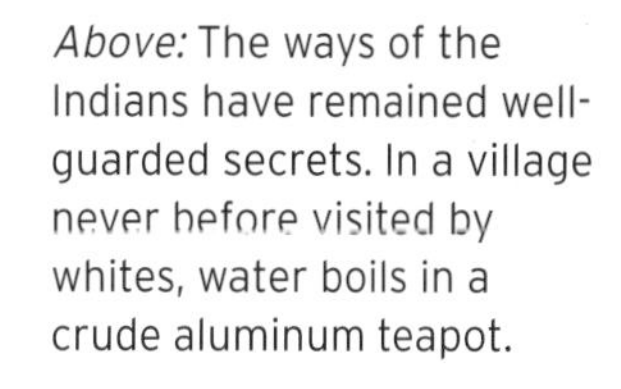

Above: The ways of the Indians have remained well-guarded secrets. In a village never before visited by whites, water boils in a crude aluminum teapot.

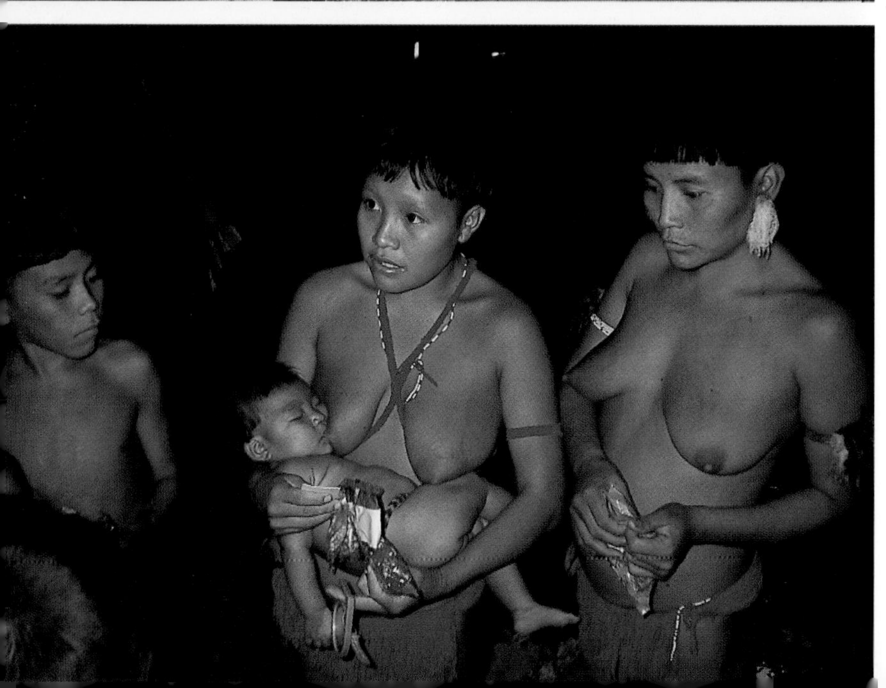

Left: The first white explorers of the region expected to see "Amazons." Instead, they encountered the ever-cheerful Yanomamo Indians.

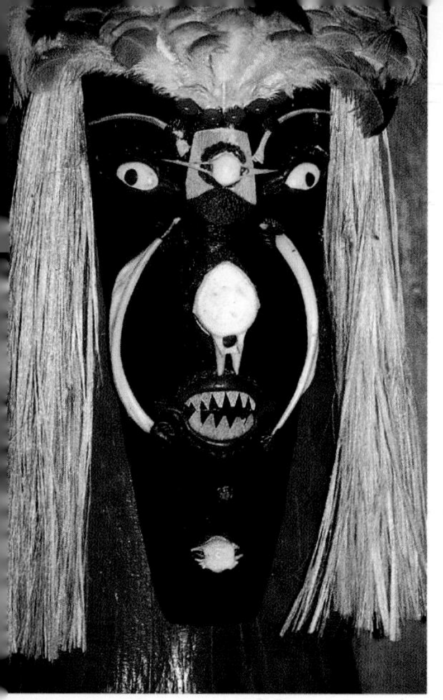

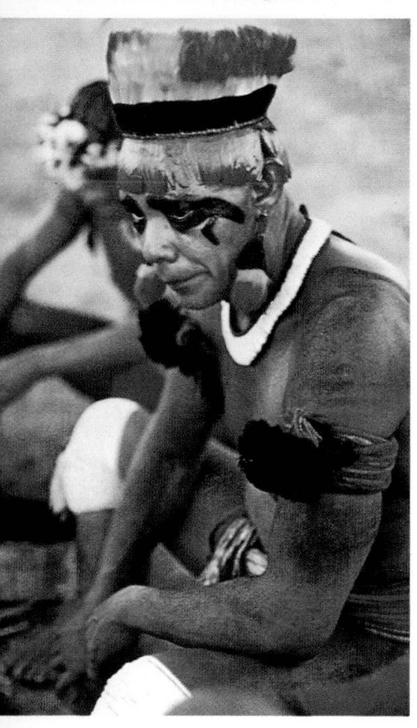

Top: Ritual mask made of bast fibers, bones, and teeth of the fearsome piranha.

Bottom: Indian from Rio Xingu takes part in a ritual.

The destruction of the rainforests also threatens not just the development of natural medicine, but important elements of our food supply as well. Cultivated forms of cacao, vanilla, cinnamon, palm oil, bananas, avocados, and mangoes are only copies of the originals, which "hang" in a worldwide museum that spans regions to the north and south of the Amazon Basin. If one of our cultivated forms falls prey to pests or disease, access to the original variety is essential to survival of that species.

Just as researchers of the cosmos are reasonably certain that there are many planets beyond our solar system which must be similar to our own, the botanist assumes that in the rainforest there are thousands of plants which are totally unknown to us, copies of which could enrich our food supply—unless, of course, they are put to the torch in their first encounter with humanity.

I have often lain in my hammock, in a semi-conscious state, reflecting upon the power of the rainforest to survive. My mind's eye has taken me on walks with my Indian friends; we have seen heavenly rainbows, and I have thought, as they do, that it would be a crime to lose one single leaf. If we lose one, we run the risk of losing everything. For the Indians, the rainbow is at once a shimmering sign of the magnificence of heaven, and visible proof of the truth of the beliefs that have been handed down to them.

After such mental journeys I awake again, fully conscious, and realize that all green things are engaged in a struggle against their environment. They seem to have mastered every natural obstacle or threat which faces them—the rapid currents which threaten to carry away the very soil that supports them, floods which reach the highest leaves and transform tall jungle trees into underwater plants. They also must overcome the eternal twilight of the deepest rainforest, and must grow to a height of at least fifteen meters before they can receive just a few meager rays of sun. Must all of this be destroyed?

At our first meeting, my editor said, "Don't write an appeal for the preservation of the rainforest. That's another book, and the discussion should take place elsewhere."

I've tried my best to follow his advice. My hope is that after reading the following chapters, readers of this book will feel that such an appeal would have seemed superfluous. If this book can communicate new knowledge on the healing powers of plants, as well as provide arguments in the debate for the survival of the rainforest, I will have done much more than to have fulfilled my mission.

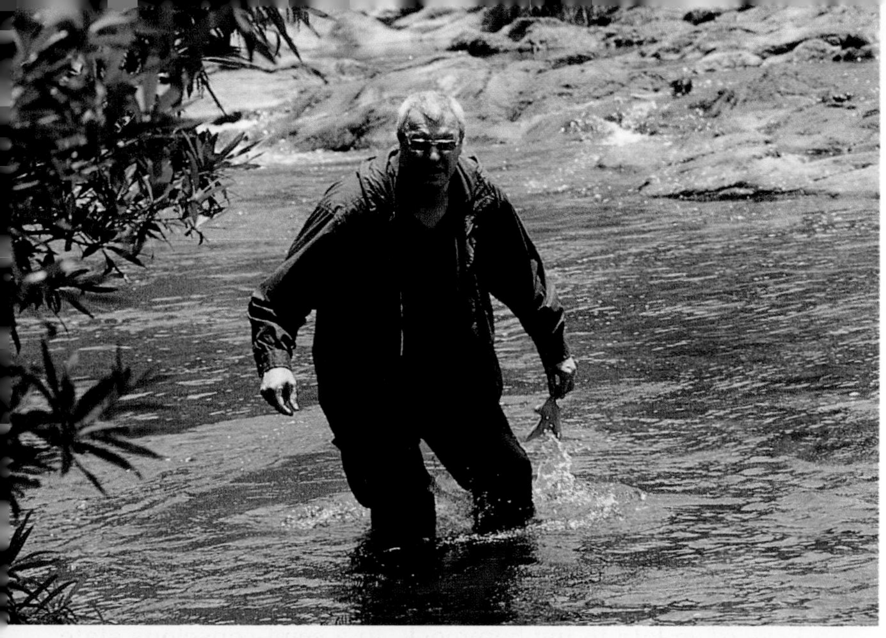

Left: In danger near Barcelos. A sudden rain can turn large tracts of land into lakes overnight.

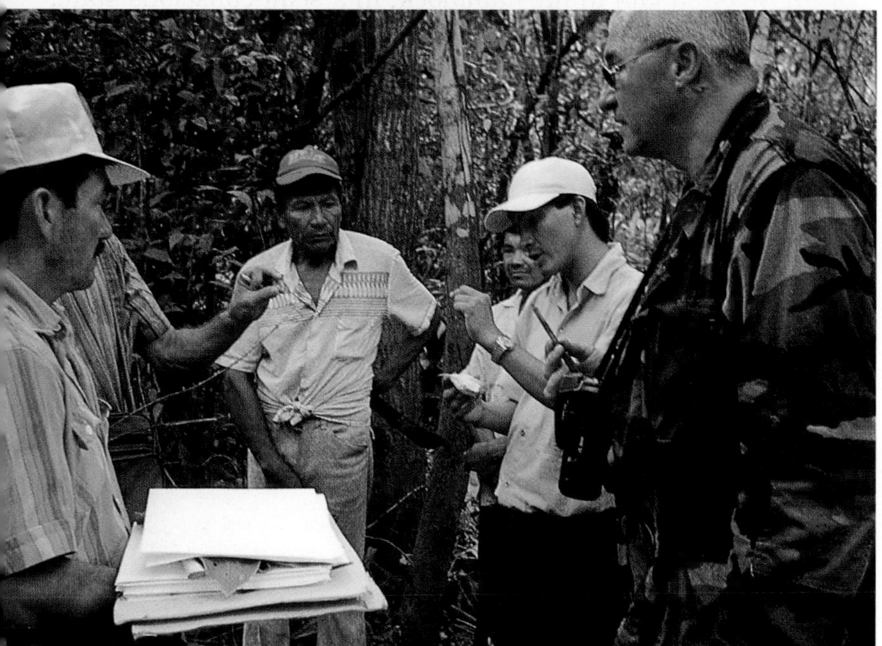

Center: A "workshop" in jungle plant medicine. A team of helpers guarantees a steady supply of CoD Tea.

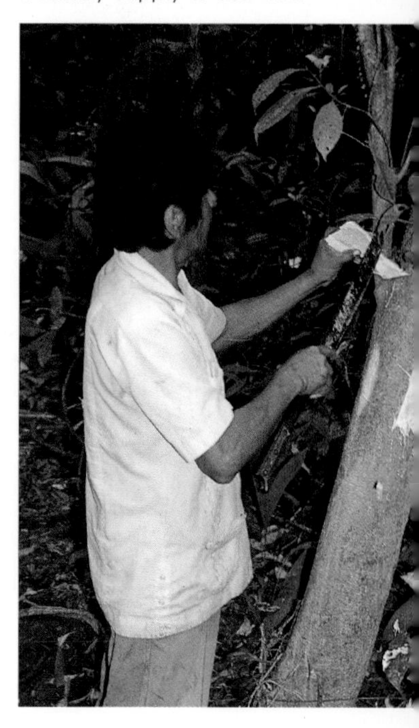

Above: The Indian diet consists of fruits, vegetables, fish, and certain leaves, roots, and tree bark.

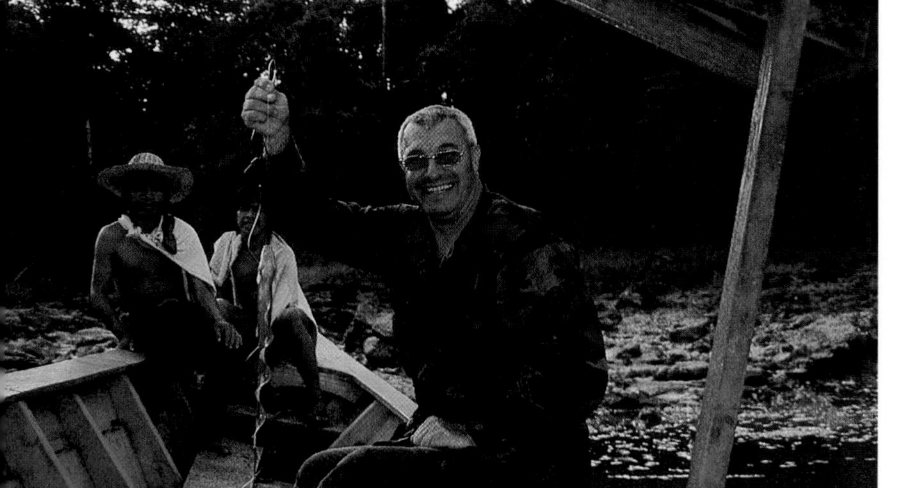

Left: The rainforest is no bread basket. Countless explorers have starved to death in the green jungle. Skill in fishing is essential for survival.

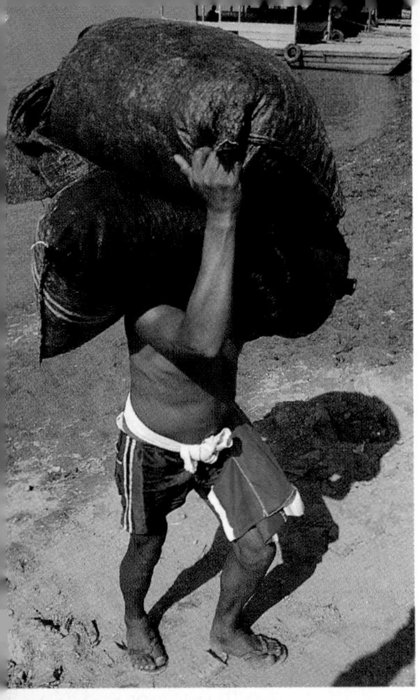

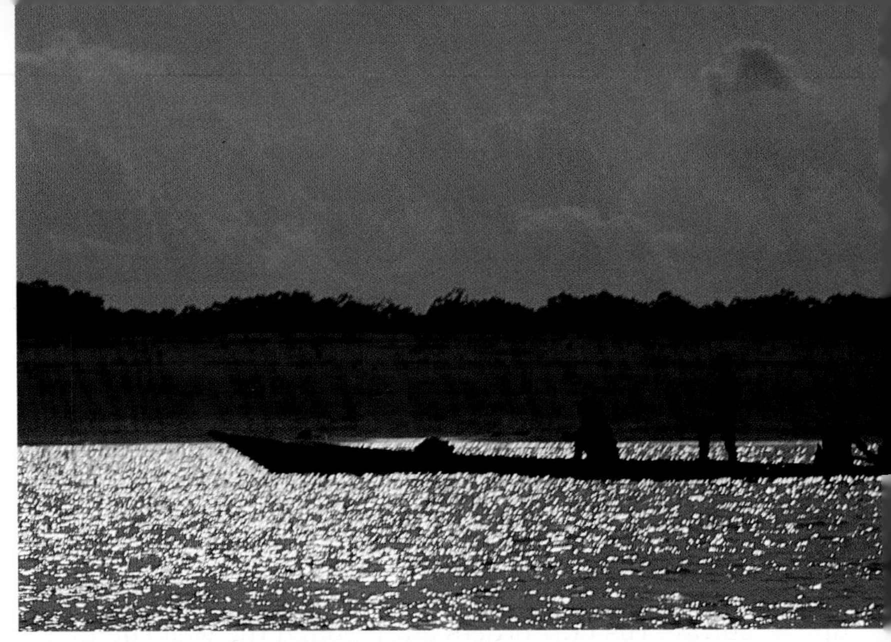

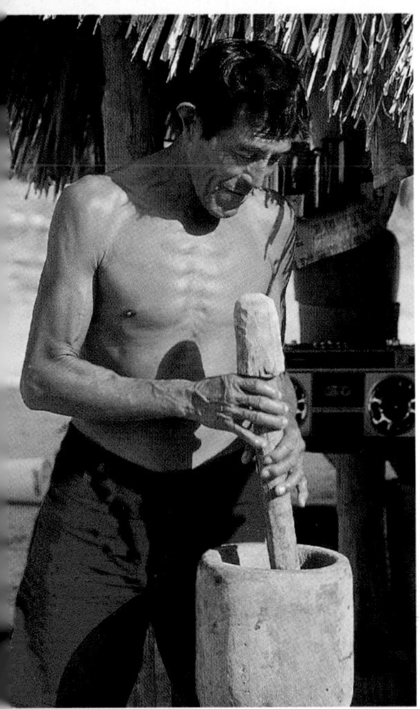

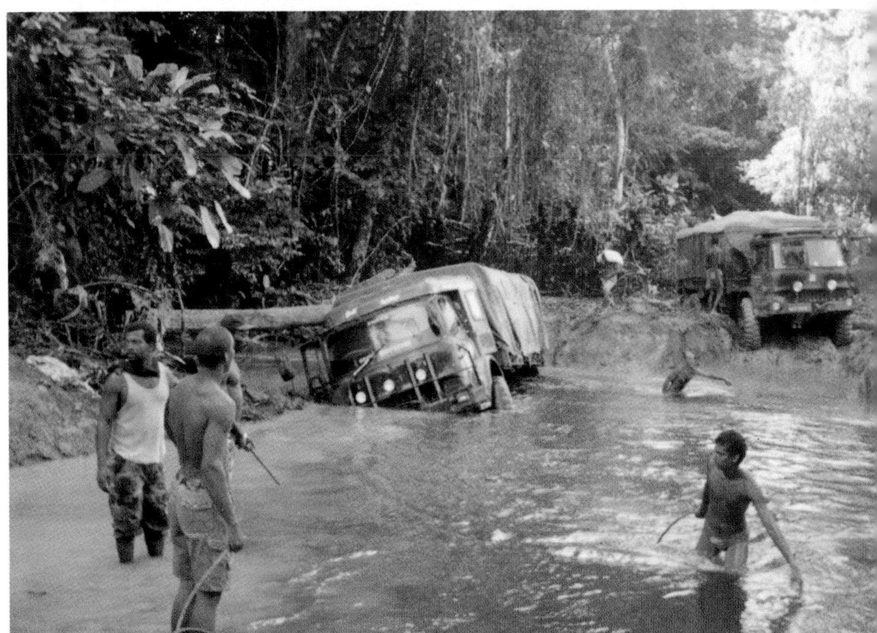

The ingredients of CoD Tea are gathered and processed by Indians. They are then transported by foot, then by canoe, and then by truck for more than three thousand kilometers to the Atlantic.

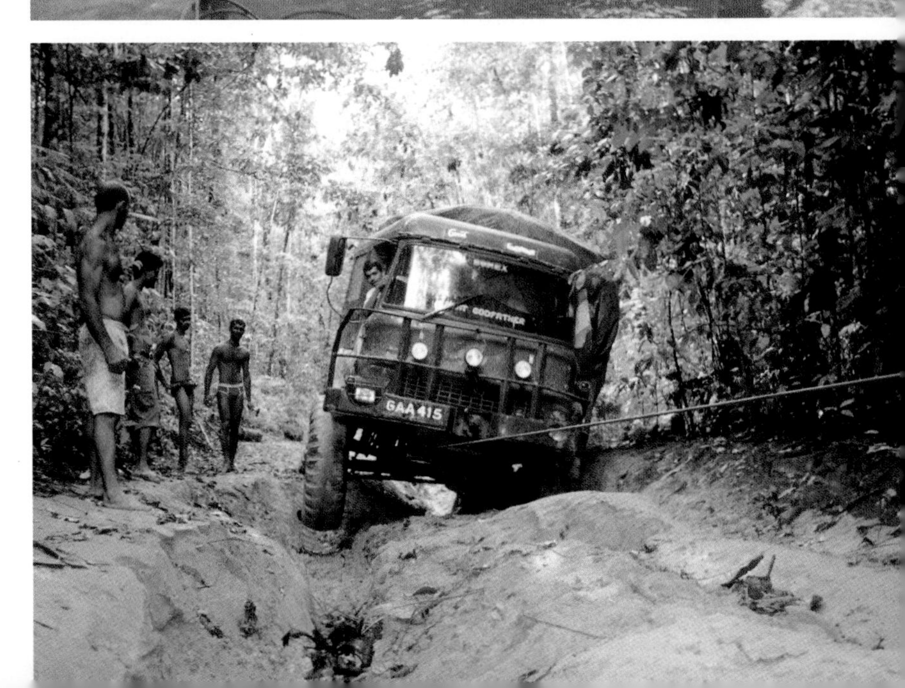

A Strange Reward

The hip operation on the young Indian boy at the orthopedic clinic at the University of Sao Paulo was coming to an end. Dieter, the visiting surgeon from an upper Bavarian valley between Bad Toelz and the Karwendel Mountains, began closing up the suture. His curt orders cut through the well-equipped operating room as his delicate hands carried out movements practiced thousands of times before. The scene would have made a TV director happy.

What a director probably would not know is this: surgeons and nurses react on such an occasion as anyone would when the hardest part of a job is over and the finish line is in sight. The adrenaline level drops, the nerves begin to relax, and muscles over which we have no control decide to take a break.

All over the world, surgeons are especially wary of this state of reduced concentration. If sloppy mistakes do occur during an operation, this is the time. I often picture myself as a pilot at the tail end of an eight-hour flight over the Atlantic who has to land safely in New York or Rio. I notice that Dieter uses another method. His orders become louder, almost sharp, which gives the scene an almost dramatic touch.

I was present only as a technical adviser, and did not worry much about Dieter's technique of sharpening his concentration at the end of the operation. My nerves were playing Pavlov's dog with me. In the midst of the smells of chloroform and disinfectants, I suddenly smelled the aroma of fresh-roasted coffee, as it is found only in Brazilian hospital canteens. I headed toward the canteen. Dieter would catch up with me later.

If only for the pleasure of having been introduced to Brazilian coffee, my trip to Brazil would have been worthwhile. I had been invited by a Brazilian to give a lecture and demonstration on a hip replacement procedure developed by Professor Rainer Kotz, Dieter Uyka, and myself.

An 1830 lithograph. Since its first discovery by Europeans, the Amazon has been a compelling challenge for artists.

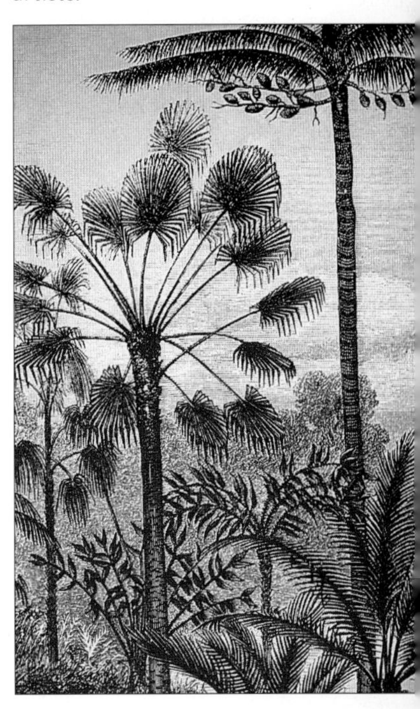

As I was packing up my slides and manuscript after the lecture, one of the attendees in Sao Paulo asked me, "Would it be possible for you to be present at the first operation?"

I agreed immediately, and he rewarded me with some fascinating stories. I am thankful to him for so much good advice, which made planning my research trip up the Amazon much easier and allowed me to return home in one piece. Until that time, I had never dreamed of making such an expedition.

I had just left the operating room when an old Indian man approached, walking toward me with regular steps and upright posture. Notwithstanding his unusual dress—torn jeans and a faded polo shirt—he had a noble bearing. His chestnut eyes were fixed on me.

"Are you the European doctor?" He was obviously referring to Dieter, so I answered, "No." But he didn't let up. He thoughtfully fished around for a newspaper clipping in his pants pocket, and showed me an article with my picture, along with a report of my lecture of two weeks before.

"I've come here to thank you. The white shaman will help many from our tribe. Women will be able to walk again, children will be able to climb. I've brought you a gift." Perhaps I should point out at this time that Asian and Indian women have a much higher incidence of the hip displacement for which our new procedure was intended.

At this, the Indian pulled out a small bundle from his belt. The four corners of the cloth were tied in two knots, which he untied, carefully opening the bundle to show me the contents: a few dried leaves and branches and some pieces of bark.

It is not common knowledge that doctors often receive payment in the most unusual forms. One of my Hungarian colleagues once received a light bulb for his refrigerator. The original had blown, and replacements, thanks to Communist mismanagement in Hungary, were impossible to find. The patient had badgered Western tourists staying at the hotels for Westerners in Budapest until one finally relented and agreed to trade a bulb for three jars of goose-liver pate.

I smiled politely at the old Indian, thinking of olive branches, nutmeg, and other symbolic plants, and was happy to receive this gesture of gratitude. The old Indian gave me such a penetrating gaze that I almost began to feel guilty because I had nothing to give in return.

A short time later I told Dieter of my new wealth and showed him the leaves, which seemed to be long past their prime. They presented a pathetic picture, sitting there between my coffee cup and the sugar dispenser. But instead of laughing with me Dieter scrutinized the leaves and bark like an Amsterdam diamond cutter examining a curious stone. He baffled me with a question, "How did you react when he gave it to you? Think hard, it's very important."

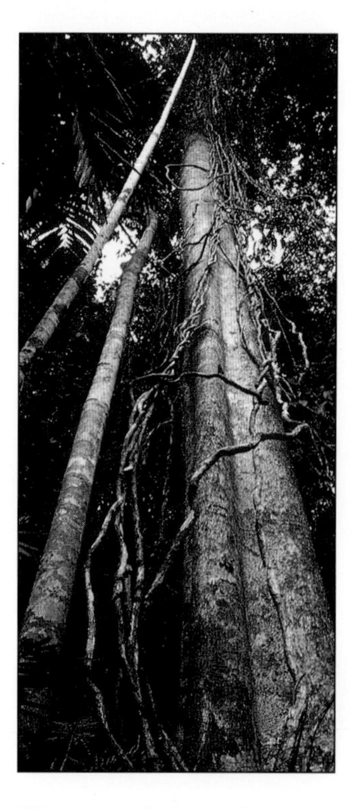

Vines come in many shapes and sizes. Some are as smooth as a copper pipe, while others are rough like rope.

The Evil Eye

I told him truthfully that I had felt somewhat bemused but was pleased, and tried to show as much.

"Do you think he noticed?"

"Sure. He was staring at me the whole time, as if I was a counterfeit bill in a wad of real ones."

"Right," said Dieter. "He wanted to know if you have the evil eye."

"The evil what?"

"The evil eye! It's not easy to explain, but I'll try. The Indians believe that envy and jealousy are the roots of murder, death, and everything evil. They don't think of illnesses in the sense that we do. If one of them falls ill, unless it's a wound of some kind, they believe that that person has fallen prey to the evil eye. I've seen it often. I have three *mestizos* who clean my house, not because I can afford three cleaning women or because I'm such a slob, no. Only one of them actually works for me, and naturally I pay only her. But her friends can't find any work.

"And now let's assume that one of the two sees the money that belongs to the third (who is actually my cleaning woman) and thinks, only for a second, 'I want that money!' Indians will notice even a passing thought like that. It's the evil eye. So my cleaning woman—more out of a desire to avoid a potentially dangerous situation than out of some noble intention—asked me if her friends could work for me as well. They share the wages.

"I'll give you another example: I go at least once a month to an Indian village not far from Manias to practice speaking the Indian language. Naturally I've become very close with some of the people there, and I always bring gifts with me. With every gift that I brought, their happiness was indescribable, but I couldn't help but notice that every gift I had brought was in turn given to someone else. It was only much later that I learned from some shaman that it was the evil eye in action.

"From then on I started bringing hundreds of little gadgets and gewgaws with me. Nothing special, but something for everyone. And I noticed that by doing this I was making everyone even happier. My mestizo house cleaners have learned about work and wages here in the city. But fear of the evil eye is something they have learned from their parents. That fear is so great that pregnant women will often keep themselves hidden for weeks at a time so no one can look at them with the evil eye and cause the child to be born handicapped."

"And if a child is born handicapped?" I asked with a terrible suspicion which was quickly confirmed.

"Then it's immediately and thoroughly examined. And if it's found unfit to live—which does not take much in the conditions of the rainforest—it's wrapped up in a bundle of leaves and left in the jungle. Hours later, it will be gone. For the Indians, it's a sad but necessary thing. It's a matter of survival, just as it was for our ancestors in Europe fifteen thousand years ago.

"I don't know if I've already told you about the Italian missionary up at the mouth of the Orinoco river. I think it was about 1968 that he secretly tried to save one of these infants. Shortly after that, they were both missing. It is probable that warriors had found out about the child and killed it out of fear that it might give the evil eye to healthy children. There is a fear that a handicapped child would not be able to play and climb and keep up with normal children, and might then give them the evil eye. Here we see the evil eye helping to promote survival of the fittest and survival of the tribe. Only the healthy can reproduce."

I didn't want to hear any more. The day had been hard enough as it was. So I said, "I'm sure I didn't have the evil eye when the old man gave me these weeds."

It seemed to be the day of the searching gaze. I was again being scrutinized by someone, only this time it was Dieter. He spoke to me in the exasperated tone of a soccer coach who is explaining to his forward for the hundredth time how to defend against a corner shot.

"Maybe you would have had it if you had known exactly what he gave you. If I'm not mistaken, and I believe I'm not, many distinguished professors, if found in similar circumstances, would look as if they were miners who had just struck

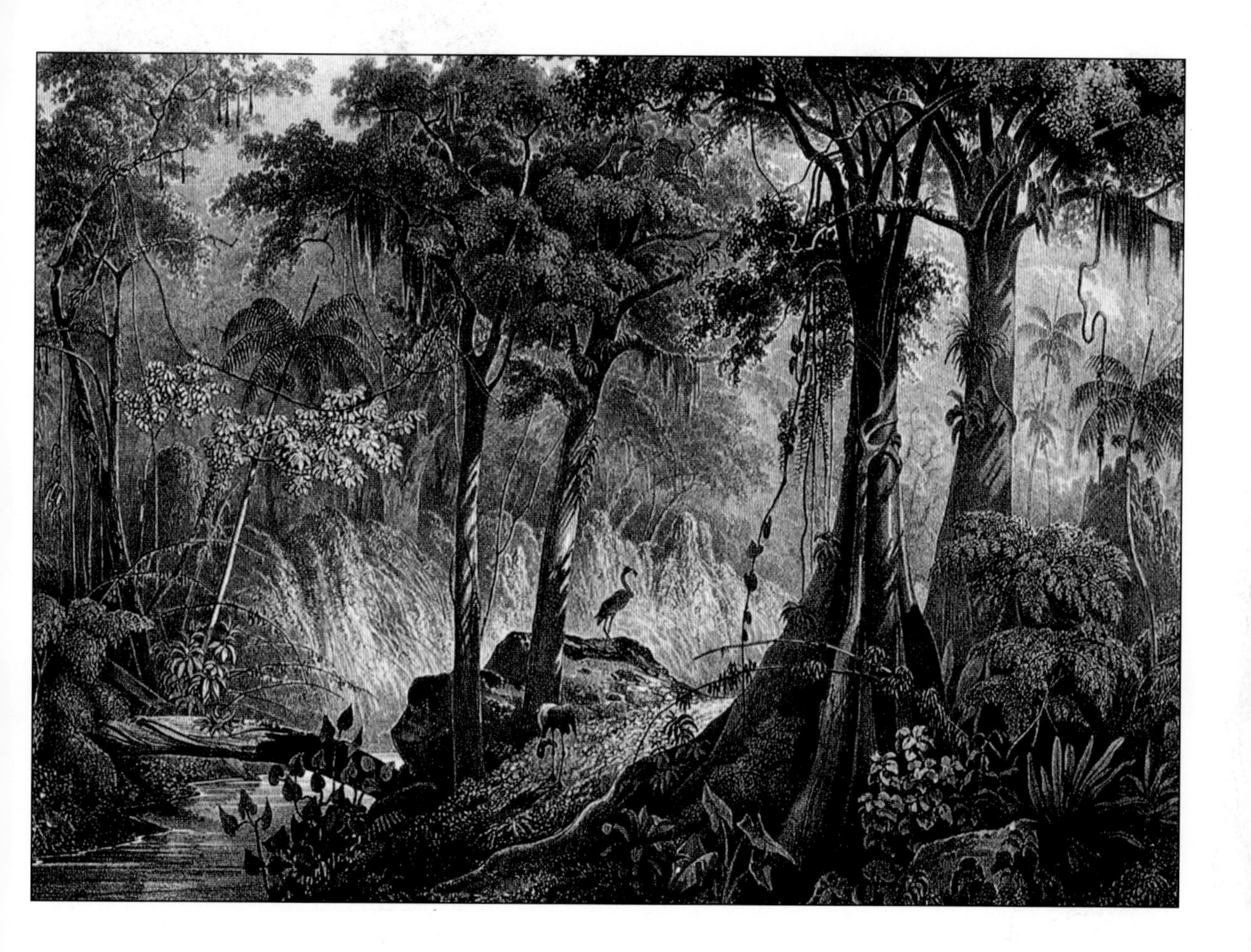

1827 lithograph from "Voyage pittoresque dans le Brésil" by a Parisian artist.

gold. What you just called 'weeds' are in fact medicinal plants, my dear fellow. Adventurers and half-baked botanists risk their lives going to the darkest reaches of the rainforest to learn something about these herbs. They hunt for shamans as if they were rare animals, with the hopes of squeezing some tidbits of knowledge out of them. More than a few shamans have been tortured or murdered."

My fatigue from the strain of the day had suddenly disappeared.

"What can you treat with this stuff?" I asked, and motioned for the waitress to bring two more coffees.

"I can't really say. I don't recognize these particular plants. But take jungle fever, for example. In the hospital in Manaus I worked with jungle fever cases. A lot of people come out of the jungle: traders, missionaries, adventurers, Indians, you name it. They've been infected with the fever, and you ask them if anything hurts. And they say "No." At first you think it's malaria.

You examine them, but you can't find anything. You bombard them with antibiotics. If you're lucky, the fever goes away. But the patient is so tired he or she can't even raise an arm. Blood tests show you that the immune system is totally unresponsive. And soon your patient becomes nothing but skin and bones, and dies a slow death."

"How horrible! It sounds like AIDS," I said.

"Yes, but it's not AIDS. Somewhere in the organism there is a virus that's wreaking havoc. We've been working feverishly on it for years, trying to figure out just what causes it, but we haven't found anything. And on the death certificate, when you're asked for the cause of death, all you can do is fill in a question mark. I think that Richard Spruce was probably also infected with it. He carried it around with him for much of his life, and in Europe they knew only that it wasn't malaria."

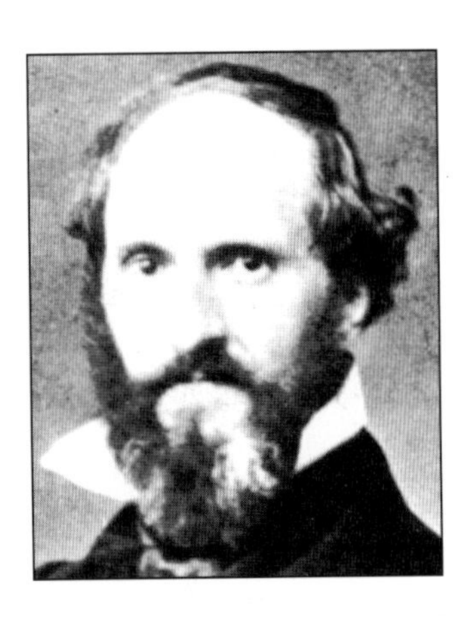
British naturalist Richard Spruce searched the Amazon region for new varieties of plants. In seventeen years, he discovered more than seven thousand new varieties.

Richard Spruce was one of the most prominent British natural scientists of the mid-nineteenth century. At the age of thirty-two he went to the Amazon, and stayed for seventeen years. He traveled again and again up and down the Amazon, gathering plants. Whenever he discovered a new variety, the British Museum rewarded him with a few pennies. By the end of his life, Spruce had discovered over seven thousand previously unknown plant varieties.

Devastated by the fever, he most probably spent the rest of his life living off a modest pension in two small rooms in his native Yorkshire. The rainforest illness had left him so weakened that he could not remain upright for more than a few minutes, and could sit up in bed for only half an hour at most. But he was able to muster his strength and resolve to finish a six-hundred-page book on his work in the Amazon, which today is regarded as a classic in the field.

"It's clear that Spruce had an exceptionally resistant immune system. I believe I've only seen one case—if that—of someone recovering from rainforest fever," continued Dieter.

"I was again in my Indian village north of Manaus. My friend had been stricken by the evil eye. It was clear to me that he was sick. I went to his hut to keep him company, but he would have nothing to do with me. I noted that in three or four weeks he had turned into skin and bones. He was running a high fever, and it seemed to be the rainforest disease. Off to the side there was a shaman instructing several Indians as they pulverized tree bark into a powder. They collected the powder in a gourd near the fire; it looked like ground coffee. I could see by their body language that I was not welcome. The next day, so as not to fall into dishonor, I worked hard at my language lesson and acted as if I had never met Raimondo before. Before my departure, I decided to pay one last visit to the improvised sick bay. I was told that Raimondo could not be spoken to, but that I could look in on him. Next to his hammock was the gourd which now contained a blackish brown liquid with whitish foam on the top. Apparently they had been using this to treat Raimondo. I wondered if I should offer to help, but saw no reason that my tablets and injections would be any more effective here than in the hospital. When I returned on my next visit, I saw that I had done the right thing. Soon after I arrived, Raimondo came to see me. His legs were a little wobbly, but he was laughing. I asked him what had cured him. He made a gourd with his two hands, led them to his mouth, and said 'Tschipo.' Tschipo is a kind of vine which grows up to one hundred meters long. The Indians use it to make rope. The drink waas too dark to have been a decoction, which would have had the color of dried out asparagus. Maybe the white foam I saw in the gourd came from this plant, but I don't know for sure. I only know that Raimondo had made a complete recovery."

"Did you speak to the shaman about it?" I asked, and ordered another round of coffee.

"I would have liked to, but he was nowhere to be found. At least I wasn't able to find him anywhere."

"Maybe on your next visit."

"There were no more visits. I made the trip, and brought lots of presents with me, but the village had disappeared. The Indians had moved on. I made several attempts, but couldn't find them. My guess is that the shaman had convinced them to move on. It must have had something to do with me; almost everything I had ever brought to the village was lying there neatly in the sand, where only a short time before there had been a village fire. The message I got was: 'We want to have nothing more to do with you.' I'm still not sure what I did wrong. I had spent two years trying to earn their trust, and now someone or something had wiped out any progress I might have made. I don't know if it was me or not."

Here Dieter paused as if he was mourning the loss of his friends. I tried to figure out why an entire Indian village would simply disappear, as if a greenhorn like me could come up with

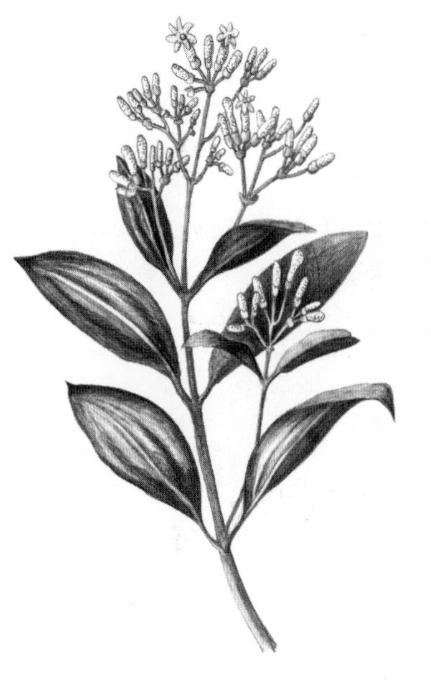

Quinine is derived from the bark of the cinchona tree. It proved a lifesaver for Richard Spruce.

a plausible answer to a question that Dieter had been pondering for years.

Finally, I asked him, "So, if these really are medicinal herbs, what should I do with them? "

"I'd say you should ask the old man. He'll probably be back tomorrow to visit our young patient."

A Remarkable Cup of Tea

The days came and went, my departure drew nearer, but the old man didn't show. Finally Dieter said, "You can't do anything with those plants in your hotel. Why don't you come over to my place tonight, and we'll make some tea. I've been able to determine that you have leaves from three different plants, and some kind of tree bark. The right mixture must have a little bit of each; we probably won't die if we try."

I wasn't so sure. Dieter just laughed, and mentioned that in addition to studying medicine, he had also gone to pharmacy school, and knew what he was doing. I decided that the chance that we would be risking a double suicide was minimal, and hours later we found ourselves in his kitchen, watching his teapot boil. The three cleaning women sat as if entranced in front of the television in Dieter's living room.

"Why don't we ask them," I said. "Maybe they know something about this stuff."

"Can't do it. To them, I'm a great white shaman with powerful magic. If I were to ask them such a question, they'd lose

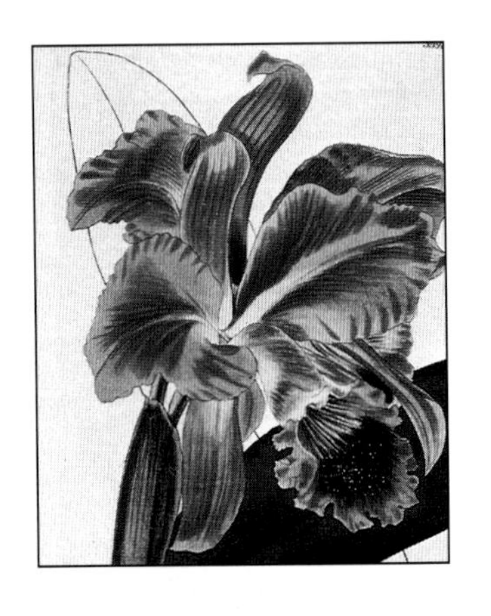

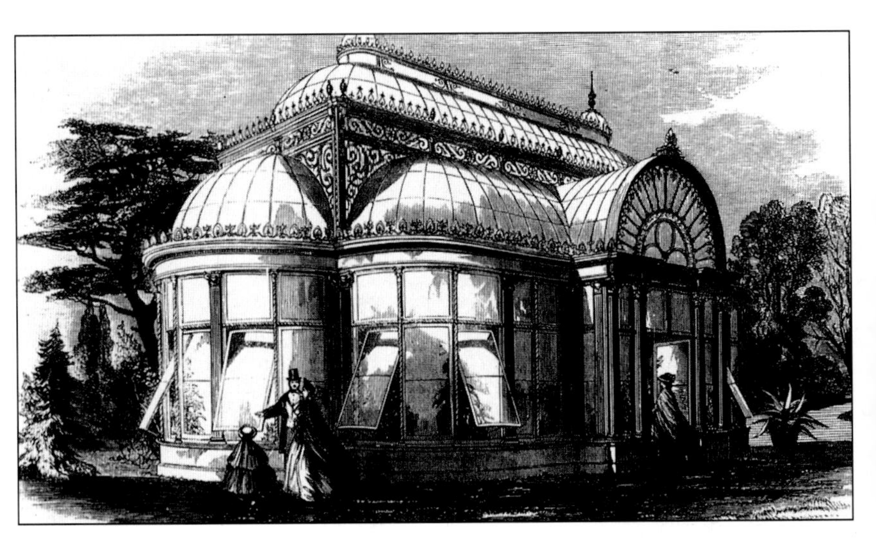

Orchids became a status symbol in England in the early 1900s. Architects made fortunes designing and constructing "winter gardens" for roofs and terraces.

their respect for me and, even worse, they'd ask me for a raise."

"But don't you think we should at least know how much we'll need to use to make the tea?"

"Please, a little more or less of one or the other isn't going to make a bit of difference."

With these words, Dieter took a large portion of the dark brown leaves, took half that amount of the other dark brown leaves, and topped it off with a handful of light brown ones. Then he took a cutting board and a grater and began to grate a piece of the bark. It sounded as if he were a blacksmith filing a piece of raw steel. In a few minutes, Dieter had grated enough for a pinch of bark dust. He tapped the powder with his index finger into the boiling water. I believe that the small amount of the last ingredient was due less to the proverbial caution of the pharmacist than to the remarkable toughness of the bark.

"How long do you think we should let it boil?" I asked.

He grabbed a bottle of Rioja, and amazed me with an estimate, the precision of which left nothing to chance: "Until this is empty."

Our senses somewhat dulled from the red wine, we took our first sips of the concoction that Dieter called "tea," which had taken on the color of a soup with nine parts soy sauce and one part water.

My taste buds, still used to the velvety taste of the Rioja, freaked at the first contact with this liquid, and sent a message to my nerve center: *Spit it out! Now!* Somehow, I was able to suppress my reflexes, and I swallowed. This scene repeated itself several times. After about ten minutes, Dieter said, "Do you feel it? It's kicking in!"

Suddenly, I noticed it, too. I galloped across the kitchen, had no time to answer the cries of the three cleaning women, and found sanctuary in the house's smallest room, where I spent the next fifteen minutes trying to rid myself of a substantial but painless bout of diarrhea. Behind the door, Dieter queried in a sympathetic tone about my "results." Suddenly, his voice took on a sharpness which was unusual for him.

"Let me in!" he cried.

Then his tone changed again. "Are you going to be in there much longer?" He was crying like a child at the dentist.

No doubt about it, the tea had had a much different effect on Dieter than it had on me. "He's getting high," I thought. He couldn't even hold a normal conversation. When I finally

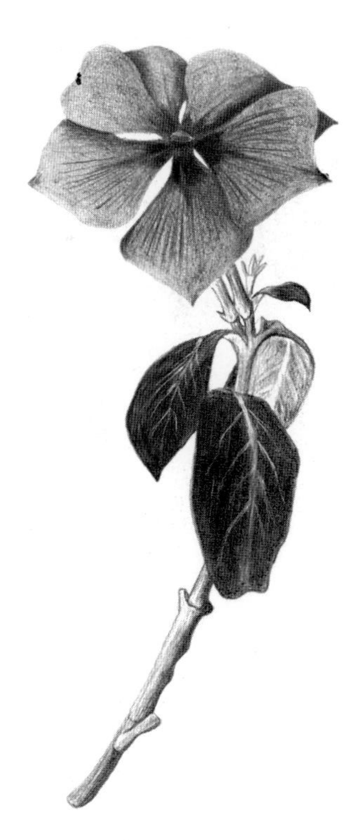

In 1962 scientists developed an extract of *Catharanthus roseus*, Madagascar Periwinkle, as a treatment for leukemia.

answered "Yeees," he answered that he needed to go someplace green.

"I have to go out in the yard."

He didn't say that in the tone of voice of one who wants to frolic among the lilies and roses, but of someone on death row trying to get a last-minute reprieve from the governor.

Three weeks later, I received a telegram in Santos: GREETINGS FROM THE OLD MAN STOP URGENT YOU COME SAO PAULO BEFORE RETURNING EUROPE STOP DIETER.

As I sat a few hours later aboard an airplane headed to Sao Paulo, I had no idea that this episode would drastically change my life for the next several years. It would lead me to the far corners of the Amazon Basin, where we would work as a team to transfer medical technology and knowledge from the shamans of the rainforest to Europe.

To this day more than sixteen hundred terminally ill patients with brain tumors, throat cancer, lung cancer, stomach, bladder, and intestinal cancer, and prostate and uterine can-

Prince Maximilian on an expedition to Brazil. 1815 copper etching.

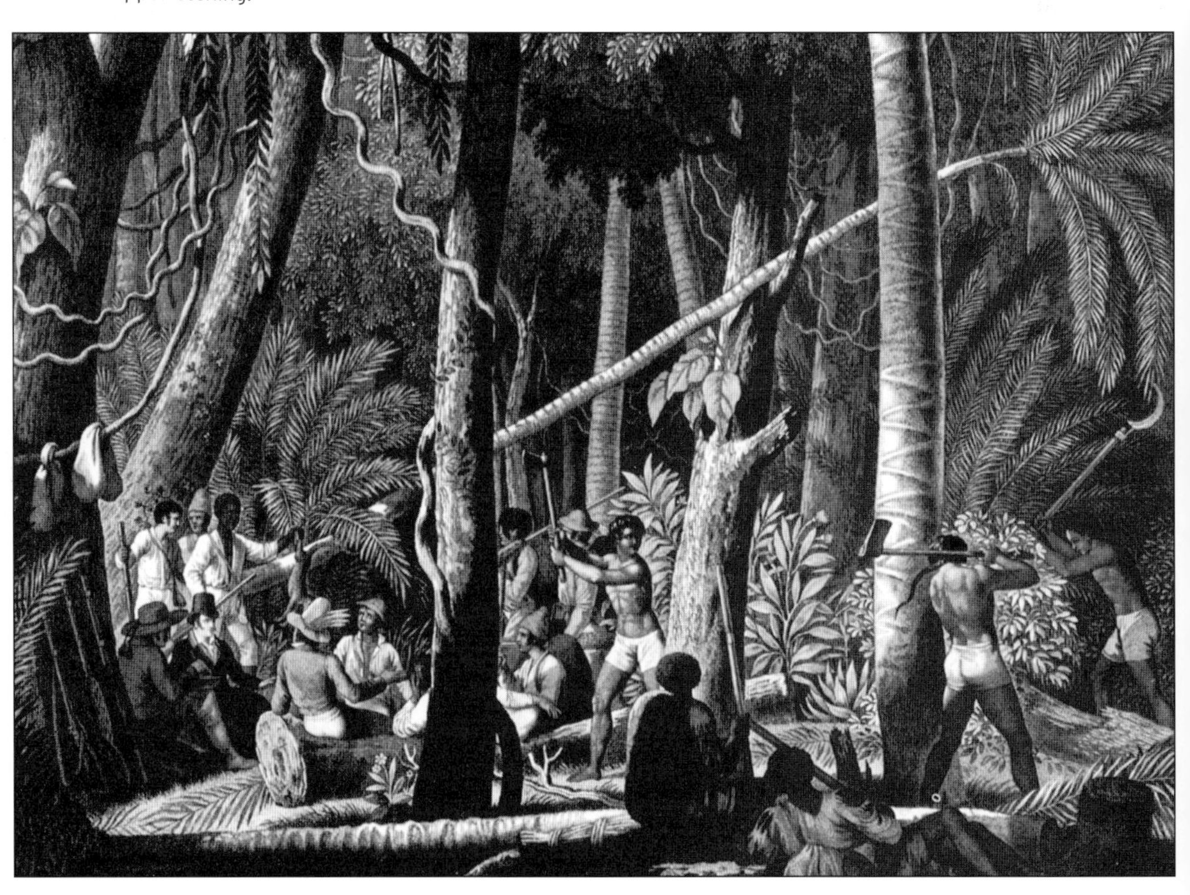

cer have been thankful for the chance to prolong their lives and increase their feelings of health and well-being to levels hardly discernible from those of a healthy person. Only the unfortunate shortage of funds, which has threatened the continuation of this program, has proven to be persistent. In contrast to most of my colleagues in research, I also struggle with the duties of an "Import/Export Manager and Purchasing Manager."

Sixteen hundred patients must be supplied monthly with approximately one thousand kilograms of tea. Indians in the rainforest must be paid promptly in cash for delivering plants. They don't accept letters of credit, checks, or barter. And it has even been necessary to explain to them the concept of work, for which they have no word in their language(s).

Pater Stipe, a missionary from Dalmatia, has given me inestimable assistance. He was firmly convinced that it would be best for the Indians never to come in contact with the outside world, but after years of doubt he has come to the conclusion that that is inevitable and cannot be avoided. He has also concluded that the Indians should be as well prepared for this contact as possible.

"In meeting the challenges of daily life, they are superior to us. They see better than we can, they hear better than we do, they can discern in an instant whether something hanging from a tree is a strong vine which can be safely grabbed or a snake that will react dangerously to the slightest movement. They know where you can cross a river, and where you can't because piranhas may be lurking nearby. They know which currents will carry you, and which will drag you under. And they get the short end of the stick anytime they have any dealings with gringos. The result is that they mistrust the gringos, that they hate them and will kill them, and that they themselves are hated and killed."

Pater Stipe became convinced that it was unavoidable that *his* Indians would eventually come into contact with the outside world, and that they could be of some use if they learned the concept of work. He had them cut wood, and they would never work for more than an hour, but it was an hour all the same. For one hour of work, he would pay them in lipstick they could use for body paint, or a roll of peppermint candies, or some other sign of his appreciation. Eventually, they began to develop a very loose notion of the relationship between work and wages.

From 1815 to 1817, Prince Maximilian, a great admirer of Alexander von Humboldt, explored areas inland from the Atlantic coast of Brazil. His reports of Indian encounters were remarkably objective compared to those of many writers of the time.

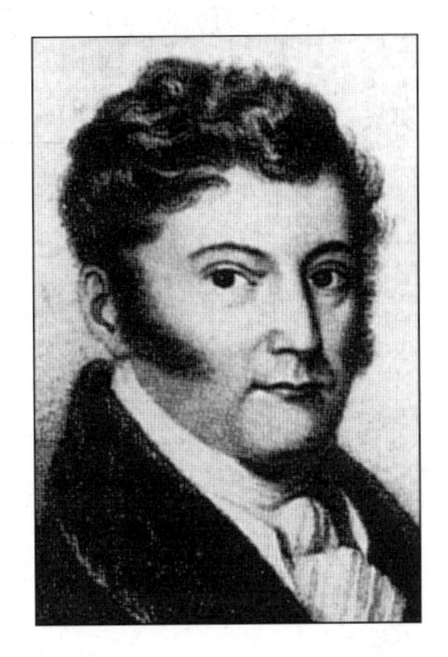

For me and for the patients in Europe, Pater Stipe's work has been a godsend. I would ask the Indians what they needed, and would explain to them which plants we needed in which amounts. I agreed to pay them when we received delivery of the goods.

Besides the punctual payment of the Indians, we needed to

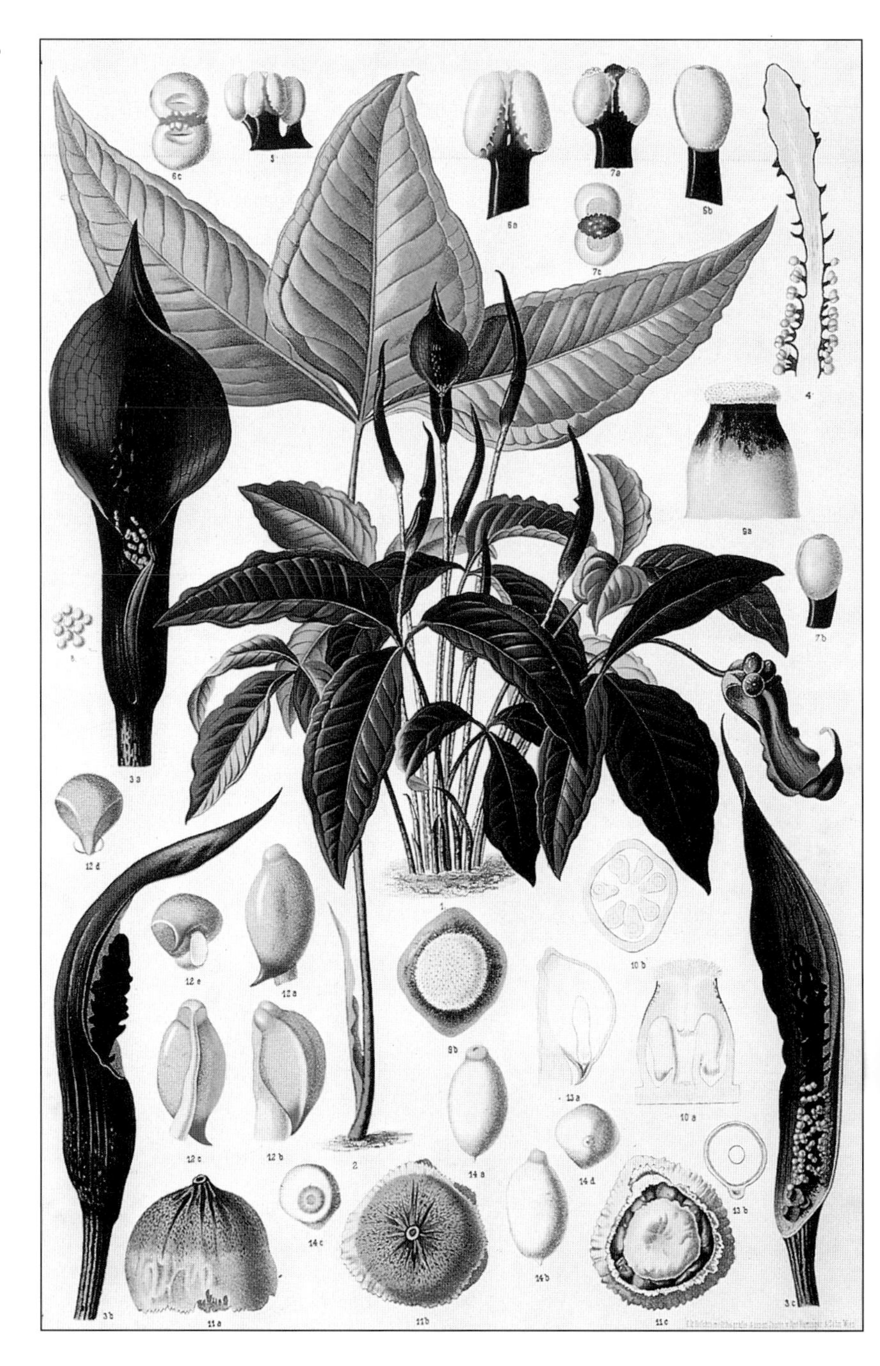

A page from *Aroldeae Maximilianae*, a major botanical work from 1879, in which a scientist and artist worked together to develop a systematic means of classification. Most botanists of the time were skilled artists.

develop an extensive distribution system. More significant, it has been important to keep greasing the wheels of that system. Perhaps most daunting have been the transportation costs. The plants have had to be shipped by airfreight, because they would spoil if shipped by sea. That the distribution and shipment have gone smoothly despite all these hurdles, I can only attribute to a miracle.

Manaus
BRASILIA

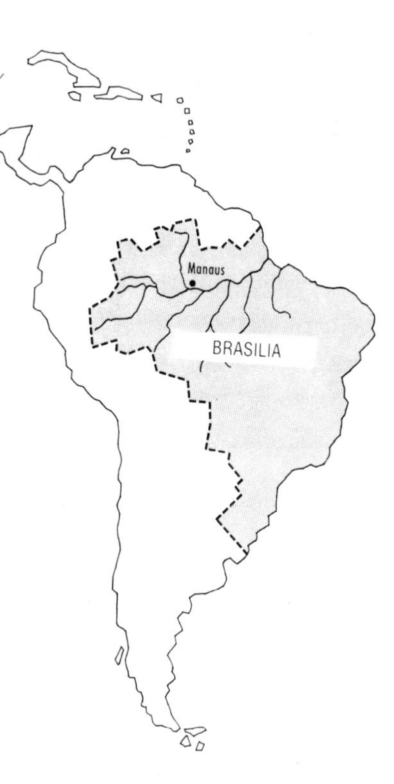

The Amazon: Terra cognita and terra incognita. At its source, the river flows to the west, but when it reaches the southern part of the continent, the Andes stand in the way. The river "changes direction," and flows to the east.

A DEMARCAÇÃO DA TERRA
INDÍGENA YANOMAMI
REPRESENTA A DECISÃO HISTÓRICA E
HUMANITÁRIA DO GOVERNO DO BRASIL DE
GARANTIR A UM POVO O DIREITO ÀS SUAS
TERRAS IMEMORIAIS.
PRESIDENTE DA REPÚBLICA
EXMO. SR. FERNANDO COLLOR DE MELLO
MINISTRO DA JUSTIÇA
EXMO. SR. CÉLIO DE OLIVEIRA BORJA
PRESIDENTE DA FUNAI
SERTANISTA SYDNEY FERREIRA POSSUELO
SURUCUCU-RR, MAIO DE 1992

A plaque marks the border of the Yanomamo territory.

Rendezvous in the Jungle

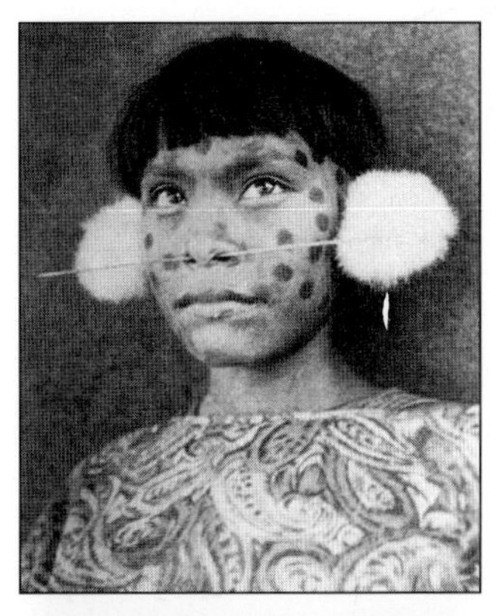

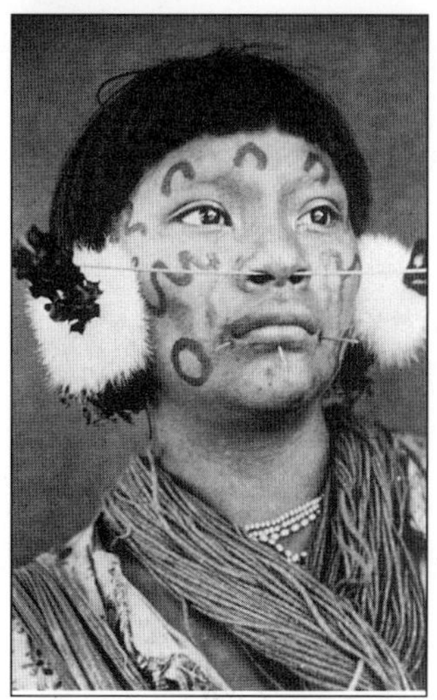

Two Yanomamo women in ritual decoration. Their faces are colored mostly black and red.

As I sat aboard the airplane from Santos to Sao Paulo, I read Dieter's telegram for what must have been the fourth or fifth time. Was it a call for help? Had there been some unexpected complication after the boy's hip operation? Since the "old man" had sent his greetings, I doubted that.

Before I had left Sao Paulo, Dieter and I kept an eye out for the old man. My departure date was drawing nearer, but there was no trace of him. When Dieter asked our young patient about him, the boy would only answer, "Katunka will be back." Dieter asked him when, and he only repeated mechanically, "Katunka will be back."

I suggested that we start looking for Katunka by checking with the hospital doorman, or at the Indian mission, or anywhere else in the city, but Dieter thought it would be pointless.

"The name Katunka is practically useless to us," he said. "It's probably not even his real name. The kid probably made it up. Indians don't call themselves by their real names. They consider the name to be a part of the soul, and it's never spoken."

I wanted to go look for him myself, but Dieter was adamant. "Forget it! When the old man hears about it, it can only hurt us. He's not going to come to us and say, 'Senhor Doctor, I've heard you were looking for me. How may I be of service?' Chances are, he'd simply disappear."

My guess was that Dieter's telegram must have had something to do with the plants which we had tested and that had affected us so strongly. I had tried to reach him by telephone, but trying to reach a surgeon who is in the operating room eight to ten hours a day is not the easiest thing. At that time, you had to go to the telephone company to make a long-distance phone call, and the fax machine had not yet been invented. Luckily, the airline was more than accommodating in changing my flight plans; otherwise, I would already have been headed out over the Atlantic toward London.

As I arrived at the hospital in Sao Paulo, Dieter was in the operating room, and would be there for another two hours. I left a message for him to meet me in the hospital cafeteria, where I would be poring over flight schedules. I needed to find a connection to London that I could make without paying a penalty, and still be able to make my speaking engagement there. As I was in the midst of this Sisyphean task, Dieter suddenly plopped down in the chair opposite me and asked, "How soon can you be on the Demini River?"

I was dumbfounded.

He continued with a jumble of names, dates, and events, which went something like this:

Two weeks after I had left for Santos, the old Indian suddenly showed up in the young boy's room. Luckily, the nurse on duty found out about it, and called Dieter, who was taking a break from his busy schedule. Dieter was able to catch up with Katunka (who introduced himself as "Mauricio") at the hospital exit. After talking about the young boy's condition, Dieter was able to bring the conversation around as nonchalantly as possible to the subject of the plants. The old man said that they were plants that the European doctor should take home with him, and that the European doctor might try to visit the Indian village before he returned to Europe. These plants, he said, can be used to make a tea used to treat the rainforest fever which plagues the gringos.

He said that his tribe should be easy enough to find: go to where the Demini and Toototobi rivers meet, then travel on foot for five days in the direction of the setting sun, and you can't miss the village.

"Tomorrow, you can meet Katunka, or Mauricio, or whatever else he calls himself, in the boy's room. He usually comes at nine A.M." said Dieter, before he was paged over the hospital intercom for the third time. As he left he said, "Come over to my place tonight. I have some good maps of the region, and we can talk some more."

Dieter assumed that I would accept the Indian's vague invitation. It was astounding. This wasn't going to be a stroll in the park. I would no doubt be traveling for weeks, and it was very possible that I would never even find the village. Nonetheless, I bought a map; it couldn't hurt to go into this with at least some knowledge of the area.

At first, it all looked so clear-cut on the map, which was a

"Mapa Politica, Escala Aproximada 1:2.270.000." Simply move your finger about twenty centimeters from the jungle city of Manaus to the city of Barcelos. There, several wavy blue lines marked the juncture of many smaller tributaries coming off of the Rio Negro, which could easily have been overlooked. If you found the place where the Rio Araca branches off of the Demini River, it couldn't be far to the mouth of Rio Toototobi. The problem was, none of this was marked on the map.

I made myself at home in Dieter's apartment. The man of the house was not in, and the three Indian cleaning women sat in front of the TV as if they hadn't moved since my last visit weeks before. They weren't bothering me, but apparently I was bothering them. Behind the television there was a bookcase with a twenty-three-volume Brockhaus Encyclopedia.

"Let's take a look," I thought, and thumbed through volume two. "Demineralization . . . Deminutivum . . . Demirel . . . ," I found nothing under "Demini River." Disappointed, I slapped the book shut. If the eighteen-hundred-kilometer Demini River wasn't in there, I was certain not to find the Toototobi.

Soon after that, Dieter arrived and consoled me with a bottle of Rioja. "I have aerial maps. They're pretty accurate, and I think you'll be able to learn a lot from them."

A quick look did tell me something: the area I was going to was relatively unexplored. Here and there, a hill was shown in vague contours, with the inscription "elevation unknown," or "relief data incomplete." With its thousands of strange names and labels, this might as well have been a map of the moon. But I thought at the time that a trip to the moon might seem like a weekend joyride compared to what I was planning. At this point, only Dieter seemed to be sure that I would be making this trip.

"Why don't you come with me?" was what I wanted to say, and now that Dieter was opening the second bottle of Rioja, it seemed a good time to ask.

"I'd love to come along and share the results of your exploration, my dear friend, but it's too risky."

Dieter told me that he had already been detained once for unauthorized entry into an Indian area. He had made the trip without the permission of FUNAI (Fundacao Nacional do Indio, an agency overseeing Indian affairs), the agency that issues permission for travel into Indian areas. FUNAI officials have a reputation for protecting their turf just as East German border patrol guards once reigned over the former workers' and farmers' paradise.

"FUNAI never issues permits. Or, more accurately, they simply ignore your requests. Any correspondence or requests for permission are filed promptly in the wastebasket. If they catch you going where you shouldn't be going a first time, at most you'll receive a warning. The second time, you'll land in jail, and staying in a Brazilian jail is something I wouldn't wish on my worst enemy."

What I had previously heard about FUNAI made Dieter's comparison with East German Honecker's tyranny not only misplaced, but even a bit off the wall. FUNAI was founded by the Villas Boas brothers, who were even nominated for a Nobel Prize. Along with other respected Brazilian families, they gave the organization its momentum and direction. In the 70s, however, the Villas Boas brothers resigned from FUNAI, and explained, "We are convinced that every time we come into contact with an Indian tribe, we contribute to the destruction of the purest things they possess."

Pater Stipe, the Dalmatian missionary whom I have mentioned earlier, held the same views for many years. In the end, though, he softened his convictions and attempted to help the Indians. Time has proved him right. A few well-meaning outsiders and a few thousand Indian warriors have not been able to stop the mighty wheel of so-called civilization. Indians who did not know enough to get out of the way have been crushed by the wheel. They have been killed by *garimpeiros* (gold prospectors), or infected with Western diseases against which they have no immunity.

"What should I take with me?" I asked Dieter.

He grabbed a yellowed list and read its contents like a pilot going through a checklist before takeoff: a calendar watch, compass, lighter, camera with zoom lens, small manual flashlight, hunting knife, pocket knife, pistol, cartridges, scissors, sewing needle, a notebook, Portuguese–German Dictionary, Yanomamo–German phrase book, ballpoint pen and refills, sleeping bag, hammock, malaria pills, pain killers, worm pills, Band-Aids, bandages, tweezers, tourniquet, antibiotics, cortisone, ointment for mosquito bites, mosquito netting, mosquito repellent, tape, surgical needles and thread, prostigmin (an antidote for curare poisoning), and potassium cyanide, as a last resort.

As Dieter opened our third bottle of Rioja, I said, "I'll go back

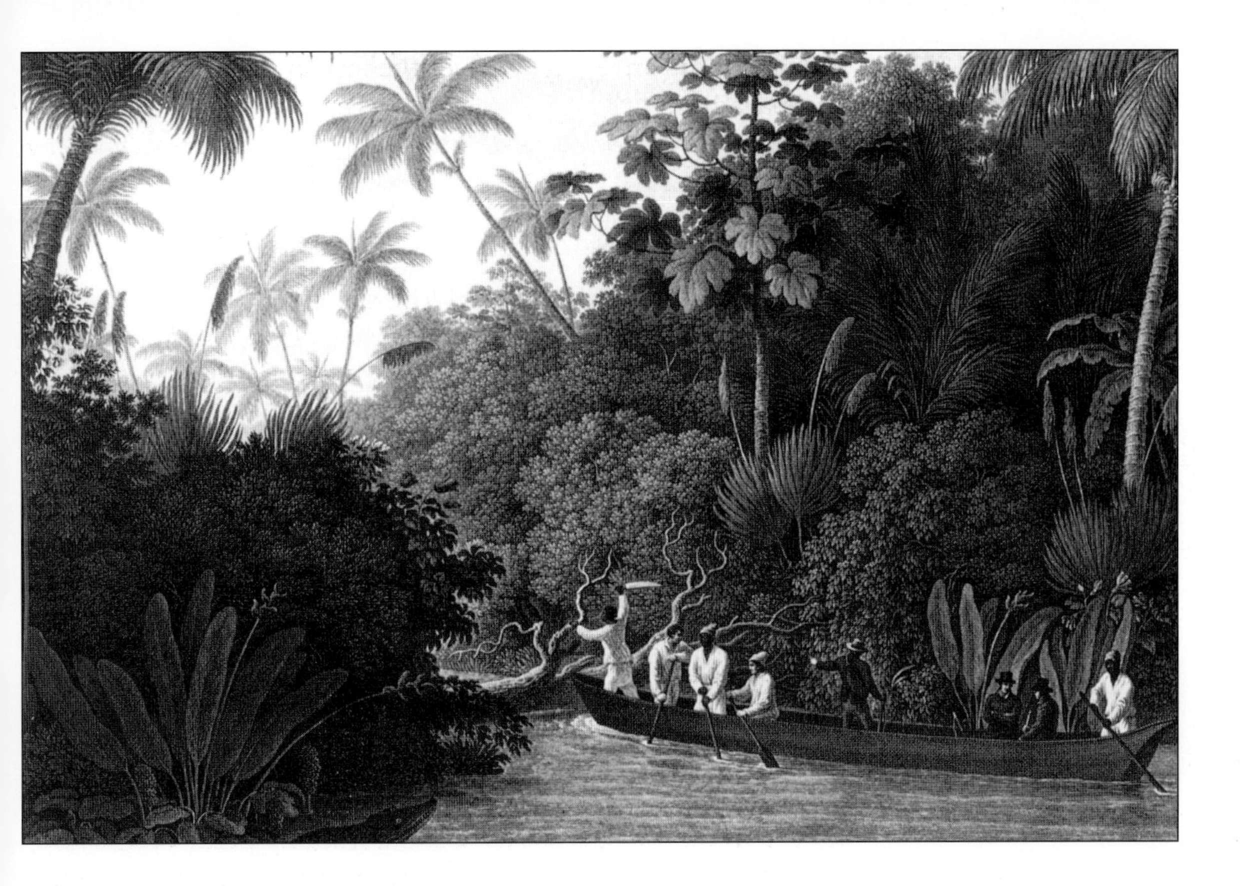

to Vienna and start preparing for the expedition." Spurred on by the wine, I continued, "I'll even fill in that missing elevation on this map." I looked at the clock; it was seven A.M.

Prince Maximilian exploring an area that today is a suburb of Rio de Janeiro. Two hundred years ago, this was all jungle. 1835 lithograph.

Planning the Expedition

The scope of my expedition to unknown areas west of the Demini River first became clear to me as I sat in the Café Landtmann in Vienna. I sat in front of my *Verlangerte mit Schlag* (thinnish coffee served with a dollop of whipped cream) and looked into the trusting eyes of my friend Peter Seisenbacher. Peter is a two-time Olympic medalist and European Judo champion. As he took a bite from a sausage (known as Wiener Wurst, but called a Frankfurter in Vienna), I wondered how may opponents must have been duped with that gentle look from those same eyes—moments before Peter dropped them onto the mat. But now, as I sat across from him in the café, Peter was squirming like a worm on a hook. I noticed it as I read Dieter's checklist to him, and came to the part about the potassium cyanide as a drastic measure to end the expedition.

"Is this really going to be that dangerous?" he asked.

"Not if we bring along a few thousand fishing hooks, peppermint candies, and lipsticks as presents for the Indians," I said as calmly as possible. This was additional advice Dieter had given me after our somewhat dramatic meeting with the old man.

The old Indian hadn't understood us, and we had not understood him. Dieter had drawn four moons on a piece of paper, two lines for the Demini and Toototobi Rivers, and at the fork in the rivers, a stick figure, which was me. Katunka, or Mauricio, or whatever he called himself, made walking movements with his fingers in the direction of the setting sun. Dieter and I decided not to let him know of our interest in the herbs.

"And what if we can't find the old man's village?" asked Peter as he wiped some mustard from his lips.

"We can't miss it. At least that's what Dieter and the old man told me."

"And you want to do all of this just because of some plants?"

Good question—one that I had asked myself often as I was preparing for the trip. Was this just about the plants? No. I had been reading a lot about the Indians since my return to Vienna, and I wanted to know more about them. But this was not enough to persuade Peter to come along. To him, this was just some trip to the jungle that easily could be put off or not even undertaken. So I told him the whole story from my first meeting with the old man, to our prolific case of diarrhea, up to my encounters with unknown and unexplored areas on the aerial map.

Once Peter had studied the inscriptions on the map, he flagged the waiter and ordered "a couple of frankfurters, please, with just a little more mustard," and looked at his fingernails. "So when do we go?"

It was May 1983. I said, "August."

"Actually, that's a fine time to stay home." Peter gazed through the window. The chestnut trees that lined the Ringstrasse were just beginning to bloom. All signs were promising a magnificent summer.

"Closing time, gentlemen," said the waiter.

"I'll pay for your flight," I said.

"For now, you can just pay for my hot dogs," he said crossly. I knew he was in.

The trip home through downtown Vienna led me past a bookshop that had ordered books and maps on the Amazon for me. I was very difficult to reach by phone, and had very little time to drop by the shop during the day, so I had persuaded a clerk to leave a small slip of orange paper in the display window if she had anything new for me.

At that time, I had invested several hundred dollars in reading material, which is not bad when compared with what I would have liked to have spent. But combing over numerous travel journals, in which various authors describe the same occurrences and the same sights over and over again, left me a bit choosy. The agreement I had worked out with the bookstore gave me the chance to study each book or map before deciding if I wanted to take it home with me or send it back. In this computer age, Vienna must be one of the last places left in the world that I could receive such personalized service.

It had become very clear to me that I must make this trip, no matter what the cost. I called Peter to arrange our first meeting, and felt a lump rise in my throat as I said, out of habit, "Café Landtmann, seven o'clock." I wasn't entirely sure I wanted to meet him at my favorite café. Here's why:

Since Konrad Zauner opened the Café Landtmann in 1873, countless revolutions have been hatched there, mighty dictators have fallen, continents have been conquered, mighty peaks have been scaled, and thunderous successes have been written for the Burgtheater (which is just across the Ringstrasse from the café). That nothing has actually come of these half-baked

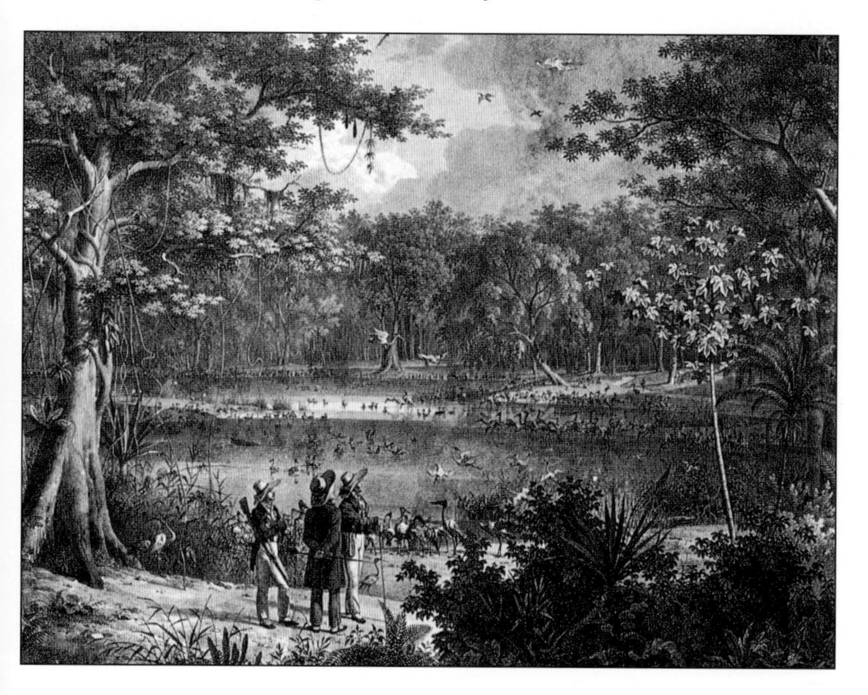

"Marsh on the Rio San Francisco."
1820 lithograph.

coups and conspiracies is probably due to the presence of Herr Robert, the waiter. His deadpan "Closing time, gentlemen" is enough to pop the most grandiose bubble, or shatter the most well-planned conspiracy. If we were to have planned our expedition in the Café Landtmann, we would have run the risk of being no better than any of the other café revolutionaries or literary wanna-bes. I had promised myself years ago that I would never belong to that group. This trip to the Amazon had become a matter of honor.

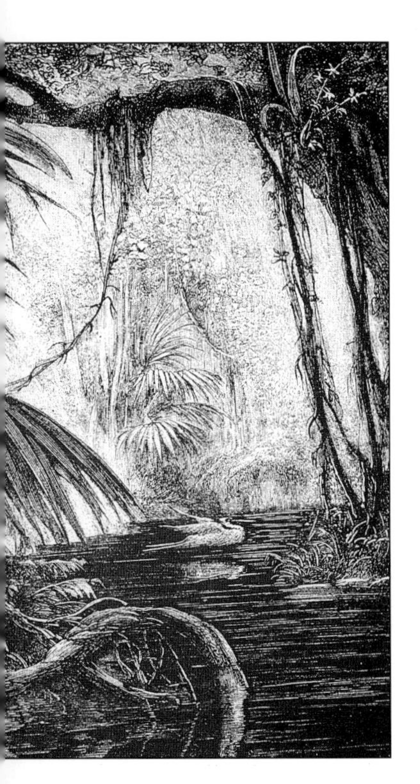

On the Rio Demini. 1830 lithograph.

Welcome Austrians

In three months, as planned, we arrived in the jungle capitol of Manaus. When I say *we*, I mean Peter Seisenbacher, Norbert Herrmann, Freddy Reichart, and myself. We were all well-trained judo experts with medals in three weight classes.

"What could possibly happen?" I thought in the comfort of the air-conditioned airport, where I was relieved to discover that all of our baggage had arrived safely with us. Minutes later, however, as the humid heat hammered us like a leg-kick and we squeezed into two taxis, I thought, "My God, what will become of us?"

Every serious author who has written about the Amazon expresses regret that they spent more time getting *to* the Indians than they did actually staying *with* them. Most had spent several weeks en route, leaving just a few days at their final destination. I wanted to avoid this at all cost, especially since my goal was quite specific. Specific? How specific were my directions? "Just go five days by foot west of the juncture of the Toototobi and Demini rivers to a place where another river may or may not branch off, then head through the jungle for four days (or fifty kilometers, whichever comes first)."

More than ever I considered this trip a chance to learn as much as possible about the plants the old man had given me. We decided to allow ourselves only two days in Manaus to get used to the climate, and then take a boat 750 kilometers up the Rio Negro to Barcelos.

We spent our two days in Manaus, putting on an impressive display of rampant gringo tourism. We bought sun hats, hammocks, and mosquito netting. Peter paid six dollars for a hand-sewn gun belt with cartridge loops. Naturally, we took lots of pictures: the harbor market, the booths and stalls in the avenidas, the cathedral, the incredibly beautiful customs house, and last but not least the Teatro Amazonas, an ornate opera house built in the heyday of the Manaus rubber boom.

Manaus was a boom town from about 1870 to 1890, and we were told that the city was so wealthy then that people would send their dirty laundry to Europe to be cleaned. Even if this is not entirely true, it makes for a good story. It may be helpful to note that the magnificent gilded facade of the Opera House was designed by Domenico de Angelis.

At the time of our visit, time and termites had eaten away at the Opera House's beauty, but since then it has been restored to its former glory. In March 1990 it began its new life with a performance by Placido Domingo as Don José de Carmen. Even Mozart is often performed there. On December 5, 1991, there was a world premiere of a choral work entitled *The Amazon Kingdom.* The piece consists of an eighteen-page fragment of an unfinished piece by Mozart, and has since been a staple of the concert season.

Considering Manaus's high crime rate, I would not advise the average tourist to roam the streets as carelessly and free of worries as did our group of judo experts. If you wander the city, you would do well to leave your valuables in your hotel and put on a torn pair of jeans. We met a woman from New York named Louise who had another "safety tip." She was alone in the city when we first met her.

"But isn't it risky for a woman to travel alone?" we asked worriedly.

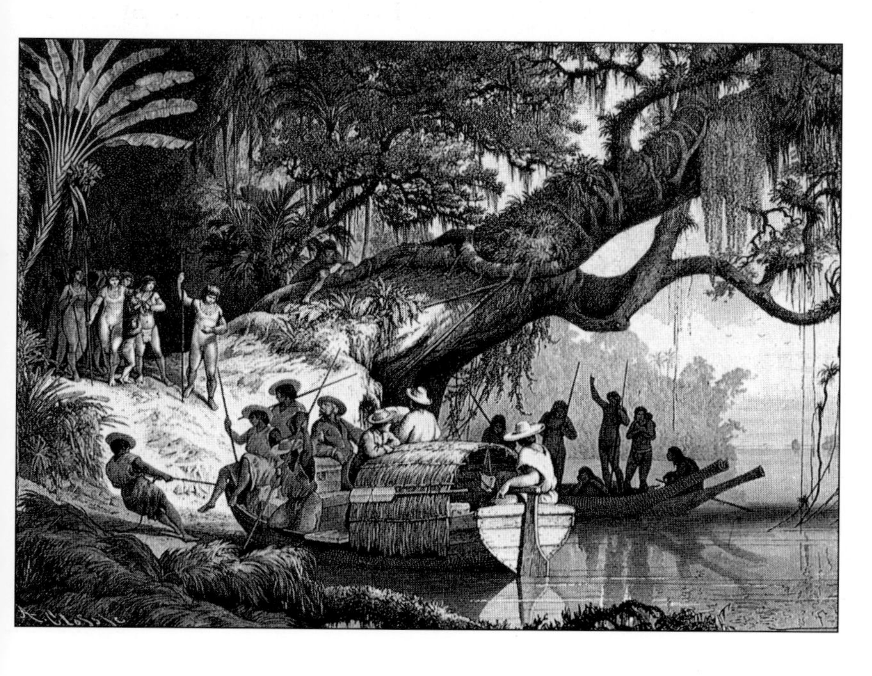

"First Encounter with Caripuna Indians" on the Rio Madeira. 1867 etching.

"I don't think so," she said. "I do just as I do in New York. Whenever I'm out alone, I just pretend to be crazy. I talk out loud, spit, twitch, and swear. Everybody stays away from me, and nobody ever bothers me. But just once I'd like to do some normal sightseeing like a normal tourist."

Our days as tourists flew by, and we were too busy to succumb to the jet lag or the 90 percent humidity. We only slowed down to buy each of us a shotgun, a .38 revolver, and 56 shells. We bought them to use only in an emergency, and did not find it comforting when the salesman handed them over the counter to us as nonchalantly as a baker would hand over a loaf of bread.

Heinrich Harrer's book *Among the Xingu Indians* begins with the following: "Better to die than to kill an Indian." Harrer made his trip into the jungle unarmed. I had read more than once, however, that the Yanomamo consider anyone who is unarmed to be an outcast from society and worthy of being shunned. Since we four Judo experts were not up to the task of being ambassadors of peace like Heinrich Harrer, and since crocodiles tend to judge all humans equally harshly, we decided the guns were absolutely necessary.

Now we could board the *Emerson Madeiros* and begin our journey in earnest. Two things I'd like to note. First, the verb *to board* reminds me of an apocryphal story:

Helmut Kautner, an infamous, much-feared, much-hated, and well-loved director of Vienna's renowned Burgtheater once cast a young and inexperienced actor in one of his productions. During a rehearsal, the actor asked him, "Herr Kautner, from which side do I make my entrance?" And Herr Kautner barked, "You don't 'make an entrance,' you simply walk through the door on the left." So I should say that we didn't "board" the ship, we simply got on with hundreds of others.

Second, the journey started with something eventful happening at every step. First at the Café Landtmann, then at our departure from Vienna, again at our arrival in Manaus, and even at our boarding the ship and our last farewell to our white acquaintances. The trip was composed of thousands of little steps, and our guardian angel never abandoned us.

The trip on the *Emerson Madeiros* is an adventure that any well-traveled tourist who finds him- or herself stuck in Manaus should experience. The *Emerson Madeiros* is a spiffy steamer registered at six thousand tons with two propellers and, at my count, only two toilets, which seem to be constantly occupied.

One of the "rules of the road" I discovered is that it's best to avoid the enticing fare of the ship's restaurant, and to bring your own water, if you want to arrive in Barcelos in reasonably good health. These reservations aside, there were some noteworthy sights and sounds—the general hubbub on deck, where a jungle of hammocks were constantly swinging into one another, the laughing and horsing around of the passengers and crew, the bleating of goats and cackling of chickens, the magnificent sunset over the Rio Negro, and, especially, the contact with all the adventurers and nutty characters who traveled with us. I have no idea if all of them had been born with screws loose, or if the jungle had made them that way. In any case, you meet quite an array of characters between Manaus and Barcelos.

I noted an unusual status symbol that I should point out. At sunrise, I began to notice that people kept giving us pitying looks. At first I thought it was just because we were foreigners. I looked at myself and at my companions, but could find nothing that would merit this kind of pity. Then I looked more closely at the hammocks of some of the people on board. They were artfully adorned with all sorts of feathers. A bicycle bell hung from one, and several toy trumpets dangled from another. Ours looked like net bags for oranges that you find in a supermarket.

I have already mentioned that the 750-kilometer trip from Manaus to Barcelos takes about two days. For a comparison, a 200-kilometer trip upstream on the Danube takes one day and one night. From this, one should be able to measure the strength of the current with which the Rio Negro flows toward the Amazon. And this force is due to the landscape, which also lends a powerful beauty and fascinating variation. The water is forty kilometers wide in some places. In other places the jungle is so close to the rear deck or the prow that it seems as if you could reach out and grab a handful of leaves. In these places, every sound from the ship comes back in a series of several echoes, and all over the background there's the constant echo of the ship's sputtering diesel engine. As a passionate sailor, I found myself trying to mark places on the map where one could tack against the wind and tried to imagine what a thrill it must be to glide soundlessly over this mighty river.

The *Emerson Madeiros* makes very few stops between Manaus and Barcelos. Off the top of my head, I can remember Santo Antonio, Novo Airao, Moura Carvoeiro, and Marova. I never left the ship at any of these places, and have no idea if it would have been worth the effort. I have heard, however, that most of them are very much like Barcelos, only that Barcelos is somewhat larger. I had read of a Hotel Oasis in Barcelos, which is run by a German family, where it would have been suitable to spend a few days until the *Emerson Madeiros* made the return trip to Manaus. We did not, however, take advantage of the opportunity to stay there. I had decided not to repeat the mistakes of those who had left themselves too little time to stay with and live among the Indians.

Fully rested after our two nights and one day aboard the *Emerson Madeiros*, we immediately started to hack away at the one thousand kilometers which separated us from our goal. At this point, I must take the opportunity to thank the Englishman, William J. Smole. His article and book *The Yanomamo Indians* gave me an accurate picture of what lay ahead of us. I can also thank him for giving me the address of a rubber trader named Ian, from the town of Moura. Ian wrote me that at the time of our arrival he would be two days by foot northwest of Barcelos, not far from the village of Baruri, and would be waiting for us on his boat. He was to be there on business, and we would pay him to take us approximately six hundred kilometers up the Rio Negro and Rio Demini. From there, we would plod through the jungle to the mouth of the Toototobi and further on to our Indian village. Along with his letter, Ian included a fairly accurate drawing of the area, showing us how to find him. We were to walk along the Rio Negro, cross fourteen branches and tributaries, and come to a place that Ian had marked simply as "hut."

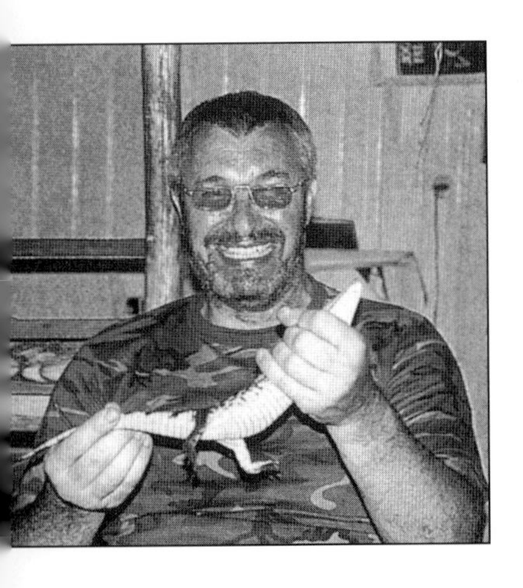

Young crocodiles have slim chances to survive. They are preyed upon by similar reptiles and large fish.

In his letter, Ian had finished with a "P.S." that was longer than the letter itself: "Because I can certainly use the money, I really want you to find the hut. I've nailed up a sign that reads 'Welcome Austrians' on the inside of the door so you can be sure you've found the right place in case I'm not there. This time of year I'm pretty busy transporting rubber from rubber gatherers. Watch out for crocodiles when you're crossing the rivers. The little ones are especially nasty. They react to every little movement, and their agitation riles the big ones, and lets them know there might be food in the area. At least that's my impression. At every river crossing, it's best to go along the bank until you find a tree to cross on, and you must secure it with vines. Otherwise, it might fall into water and you might fall into a school of piranhas, which will eat you and my money.

When you're here, I'll explain how we protect ourselves from piranhas. The trick is very simple, but it doesn't always work. Then there are the water worms [two-inch, needle-thin catfish of the genus *Vandellia*] which bore their way up into your penis. The best thing is to put on a condom, but when you're flaccid, this is nearly useless. The finger from a rubber glove works better, but that's just my opinion. Good luck."

We had gone only about three hundred paces into the jungle from the ship's landing in Barcelos when we were attacked by mosquitoes. We had already found them to be a plague on the ship, but now we realized that that had been just the front line of a massive swarm. One of the buggers bit me on the back of the hand, and I watched as my hand swelled up until the skin broke and I started to bleed, which attracted even more attackers.

We dropped everything, and rubbed ourselves furiously with mosquito repellent all over our bodies.

Norbert noticed how fat they were. "Didn't someone say, 'too few insects, no birds'? I say, 'too few birds, too many insects.'"

Freddy and I agreed. Peter, however, continued, "This is the way it is, dear boys. In this kind of heat, the birds can't be bothered to fly. So they don't go hungry, it's all been arranged that all they have to do is open their beaks, and they can feast on about two billion mosquitoes." I thought, "My God! We've only gone the first three hundred paces into the jungle, and my friends are as crazy as some of the characters on the boat."

Then I said, "The first steps are always the hardest."

My friends answered me with looks that showed me that they were thinking the same thing of me that I was of them.

After an hour, I had lost most of the feeling in my right hand from slashing through the undergrowth. The vines and half-grown scrub seemed as impenetrable as a fortress wall.

"We should probably keep a little further from the river. There are more trees and not so much sunlight, and the undergrowth is probably not so thick. It might be better," suggested Peter.

"Yeah, but we don't want to miss Ian's hut," I countered.

"That won't be an issue for some time," said Peter.

We had been under way for four hours, and had probably covered, at most, five kilometers. No, we weren't in danger of missing Ian's hut. In the distance, we heard a sound that was not the Rio Negro.

"Listen! Listen!" exclaimed Freddy, showing some signs of

exhaustion. "That must be the first tributary. Thomas, mark it on the map."

He was right. I marked our location on Ian's sketch.

In about half an hour, we came to what seemed like another river. Was that tributary number two, or just a smaller tributary of tributary number one? If Ian had accurately rendered the distances between the rivers, this must be part of number one.

"I read somewhere that a rise in the water table can create a new river," I said.

"I'm sure we'll find out. If we can find a tree big enough to cross over, it's number two. If we can't, we'll call it 1A." said Norbert.

We had a GPS (Geographical Positioning System) device, the automatic pilot for hikers, packed in our bags. But without accurate maps of the territory east of the Demini and Toototobi, it was useless.

"No problem," said Freddy, "we just walk up and down the river until we find a sign that says 'Toototobi.'"

A few minutes later, he said excitedly, "Here's a tree across the water with a vine tied around it. It must be river number two."

"Thomas, mark the map," chimed a choir of three male voices. Somewhat relieved, I made another X on the map.

"Look over there," Peter said to me in a whisper, as if by speaking too loudly he'd scare away the unusually colorful bird he wanted to show me. But when I looked where he was pointing, I saw no exotic bird, but rather six or seven fully grown Caimans, crocodiles about five meters long.

"Thank God there are no little ones," said Freddy, thinking of Ian's post script.

"We're going to need some firepower for this," said Norbert.

Three of us held our shotguns ready, while a fourth walked gingerly along the tree. Several spoonbills, great white birds, about twice the size of a stork, began to squawk, making such a racket that they nearly scared us to death. The crocodiles didn't budge, though I'm sure they had us in their sights.

All of a sudden, Norbert had this horrible black spot on his neck. I looked closer, and saw that it was some kind of leech. We still hadn't set foot in the water, but we had been up to our knees in mud. We soon realized that they were all over all of us. We stopped to pull them off one another. This was an unsettling occurrence, but later we couldn't be bothered with such trifles as leeches.

After that, we all walked single file. If one of us had to stop for any reason, the others would not break step, but continue at the same pace. Whoever stayed back would then have to rush and catch up with the others. We all had a very good reason for this system; since Manaus, we had come down with diarrhea one after the other.

"We've all had it in alphabetical order," joked Freddy. "First me, then Norbert, then Peter, and finally Thomas."

"No way," grumbled Peter. "I'm still not on a first-name basis with my diarrhea. So I figure it was David, Herrman, Reichhart, Seisenbacher."

Freddy knew better. "Just wait, and soon you'll be on a first-name basis with your 'affliction.'"

"God give us the strength to keep yammering on like a bunch of idiots," I thought. Things would be really bad if we couldn't joke about this stuff anymore, and if instead we just sat there quietly, running a high fever and gasping for air, trying to carry one another along the way.

By about five P.M. we had reached tributary number eight without major incident, and we began to set up camp for the night. We figured that we had gone just over halfway to Ian's hut. We were all exhausted and wanted to sleep as soon as we had started a fire and eaten. But all this exertion had given us energy. Like a forester checking the health of his forest, I knocked against all manner of large and small trees, and thought how much the rainforest is very much like the floors of a house. We share the ground floor with some meager plants, which can only provide nutrition for a few animals. Is that why we had seen no wildlife since leaving Barcelos, or had some disaster decimated the fauna of the area?

"Okay kids, watch out for spiders and snakes. You know the jungle is dangerous after dark."

Someone said, "Yes, Daddy."

Up in the attic, the sky was still light, but the light couldn't make it through the dense canopy of leaves. You could hear the screeching of a monkey, and other noises as well. Freed from the stress and exertion of trying to hack my way through the jungle without getting lost, I was able to hear its sounds for the first time, and tried to distinguish the different noises. A branch creaked high above me, and I looked up and saw a number of large birds. The sky illuminated them from above, giving them an almost mystical appearance. The branch rocked back and forth under their weight. Was that high-pitched whistling from them or from some other birds hidden from my view? I heard the chattering of monkeys again. Perhaps they were fighting over a place to sleep. From time to time you could hear the distant roar of some mighty animal. All this was against the background sounds of a brass concert provided by the ever-present frogs. We had actually seen the massive frogs on a few occasions. They were as big as newborn German shepherd puppies.

Everything seemed very harmless. If it had not been for the oppressive humidity, and the chattering of the monkeys, I would have thought myself somewhere deep in the Vienna Woods. Were we so blind and inexperienced that we couldn't see the dangers lurking all around us?

I had the first watch, but was nearly falling asleep as a crash of thunder woke me up. I heard a sound in the leaves, and a torrent of rain came down on us.

We crawled out of our hammocks, swore to the heavens, and proceeded to get thoroughly drenched. It wasn't exactly a warm, gentle rain, but it was an improvement on the sweat and mud on our clothes.

At first, I welcomed a thunderstorm, but then I became terrified. I wondered whether we should break camp before the rain might start a new river and throw off our orientation. But in this pitch-black night, you would have bumped into a tree if you had been standing right next to it. Freddy passed around his flask, filled with "Mama's special brew." We each took a sip and listened to the silence, and I thought, "What will we do if now there are twelve, instead of six, rivers between us and Ian's hut? And what do we do if the river overflows and we end up swimming back to Barcelos?"

Someone said, "A boat would be nice." I don't remember who said it, but I can still hear that dejected voice in my head. Luckily, from one moment to the next, the rain stopped. There was still tremendous thunder, but we slept anyway, drenched to the bone but relieved—even Norbert, who was on watch, lit a cigarette that seemed to pollute the entire jungle from the Andes to the Atlantic.

We left camp early the next morning. The rain had left us shaken. Not because we were thoroughly soaked, but because we were afraid that so much rain would change the number of rivers to be crossed and screw up our sense of where we were. To all appearances, that did not seem to be the case, although we had to wade knee-deep in water for about two hours. Even when we tried to move away from the river, the land was still flooded.

We hardly spoke to one another, and wondered now and then why we hadn't seen another living soul. Given the terrain, that was not so surprising, but we were only twenty kilometers from Barcelos. It seemed like we should run into someone along the way. Some of the guide books I had read described the area as lightly inhabited, but not totally uninhabited. Had we made a wrong turn somewhere? Was it possible that the river on our right was not the Rio Negro, but some smaller river on whose bank we would be searching in vain for Ian's hut? No, it couldn't be. We shouldn't make ourselves crazy over a couple of raindrops. As we took a break at about noon, Norbert began to shiver. The clacking of his teeth sounded like the knocking of a woodpecker.

"Can I give you anything?" I asked.

"No, it'll pass. I must've caught a chill in the rain."

I shut the medicine case, and said, "Freddy, the flask, please."

I looked at Ian's sketch again, and compared it with my map. No doubt about it, just one more river and we would be there. Soon, we had crossed it by climbing out of the water onto a massive tree trunk which spanned the entire width of the river. When we reached the other bank, we jumped into the water again. This bank seemed a bit higher than the other.

"We must be very close to the Rio Negro. I think we're almost there," I said with confidence. No sooner had we stepped onto solid ground than we were up to our knees again in mud. Harry said, "Listen!"

Somewhere ahead of us we heard a rooster crow.

We waded as silently as possible through the shallow water toward the crowing sound. We had gone maybe one hundred meters before we came to a small clearing in the forest. We saw a hut made of logs and bamboo, all tied together with vines. The flood waters had made it just to the edge of the doorstep.

We looked at one another, but didn't speak, because we knew it could be dangerous to go running into a stranger's hut in the middle of the jungle. Who knows what might happen. We might scare someone to death, or they might react in a singularly inhospitable manner.

"It's empty," whispered Peter after a while.

A ragged banner from the Holland-America Line hung limply from a flagpole. If the hut had a door, it was opened to the inside. We called "Ahoy!" and "Ian, are you there?" but nothing stirred. We walked closer to the hut. Freddy went first, and I followed close behind. We stepped cautiously into the room. Three chickens who had made themselves comfortable on the table began cackling.

"Must be the wrong hut. There's no door," I said, but Freddy showed me a slip of paper on the table, held in place by a stone.

The paper was generously covered with chicken droppings, but I kissed it as if it were my first love letter. "WELCOME AUSTRIANS" it said in thick block letters. Our most important rendezvous had been a success. What incredible luck! How often do we make a date to meet a friend in front of the opera house, and the friend doesn't show? Immediately, we become uncertain. Did we agree to meet at the main entrance or the stage entrance? You look all around, and maybe even walk right by your friend.

Here we had agreed to meet a total stranger across the ocean, 750 kilometers up along the Rio Negro, two days of bushwhacking, across fourteen rivers. If that rooster hadn't crowed, we might still be wading around in the muck.

The hut was an absolute mess (sorry, Ian), so we started to clean up. There was a fireplace, but no chimney, so we made a fire with the trash, leaves, and brush that were lying around. Before long, smoke was pluming out the window and door. Norbert wanted to gather some more wood for the fire. He stepped outside and suddenly all we could see of him was his hat bobbing up and down on the water. We discovered that a small stream of runoff led right up to the hut. Norbert came up gasping for air, Freddy said, "So this is paradise."

Two hours later we heard the gurgling of an outboard motor approaching. Before he had even reached the shore, Ian called to us, "Take it easy with the firewood. It's hard to find any dry wood."

From our correspondence, I had just assumed that Ian was English, but he set me straight.

"English? Why would you think I'm English? I'm Dutch, but that's a long story." That explained the Holland-America Line flag.

"I left the flag for you so you'd know I was here in case the damned chickens ate the paper."

"Why is it so empty here?" I asked.

"Empty? I don't know. Somebody told me in Baruri that they had seen you coming, and a rubber gatherer told me down in Tonktong that he'd seen you get your pants wet over a few crocodiles. Despite your shotguns. You could go to church naked on Sunday, and not be noticed by more people. That's what I think."

If Ian hadn't mentioned the crocodile incident, I would never have believed him. And here we had believed that no one could possibly have seen us! We had a lot to learn. Any unexpected encounter in the jungle could be as dangerous as meeting ten crocodiles.

The Dutchman seemed to be reading my mind. "You've got to be more careful. Take me for example. I could take you in my boat and leave you stranded a few kilometers upstream, take your money and your supplies, and then come back. Someone would probably come looking for you, but no one would find you. They'd ask me, and I would say, 'Oh yeah, they were here. But we couldn't agree on a price. They wanted me to take them across the river, so I did. They gave me a lousy ten dollars, but what could I do against all of them? Then I came back. I haven't seen them since.' They might believe me, and they might not."

We became very pensive, and Ian was quiet. After the last drop from Freddy's flask, he said, out of the blue, "So, anything else to take care of? Good, then let's get going. It's rained so hard the last few days that I can't get any work done, anyway." He put the three chickens and the rooster in a cage, and tossed the cage onto the boat. We threw our things in as well, and he started his motor, and we took off in the direction of the Rio Demini.

Ian knew the whole area like the back of his hand; we noticed this right away. As we were out on the open river, he sped up and a gentle breeze cooled us down. The Dutchman held onto the wheel with his left hand, and with his right reached into his pocket and pulled out some tobacco and a cigarette paper. He made a few twisting movements with his hand, and suddenly a cigarette appeared in his hand. A flick of a match on a piece of wood, and it was lit. We looked at Norbert and laughed. He had been trying for five minutes to light a brand-name cigarette with his waterproof lighter, and then tossed it into the water in frustration.

The man at the wheel began to sing, we didn't know if we should join in. He turned around and said, "What's the matter? Don't Austrians know how to sing?"

Freddy sang: "Little Hans, went alone, into the great big world."

After some time, Ian came to a tiny island in the middle of the river. There was a hut which was smaller than the one we had just come from. As we drew closer, we could see that it was no island, but a raft which was anchored in the middle of the river. As we approached, a darkly tanned man of indeterminate age lifted a barrel. He said a few sentences in indecipherable Portuguese, and Ian answered him with three or four words. The end of a tube passed from one hand to the other, and the smell of diesel fuel filled the air as we filled six reserve tanks. Ian mumbled something, the man smiled, and we were on our way again.

"There aren't too many places to refuel on the Demini," he said.

At the juncture of the Rio Demini and the Rio Negro, three freshwater dolphins jumped in front of our boat. They stayed near us, jumping and diving for some time. From the banks of the river, it must have looked as if they were towing us. Our skipper was not impressed. Nonetheless, he said, "You don't see them here very often."

I thought as much; the Rio Negro (Black River) no doubt gets its name due to its very low levels of oxygen.

The trip was a welcome rest, although we started to feel a bit guilty. Here we were, four well-trained heavyweights, fully supplied and well armed, ready to conquer the rainforest, and Ian was doing all the work. Only once in a while, he'd say, "It's okay, I'll do it." But we would soon be rid of our feelings of guilt.

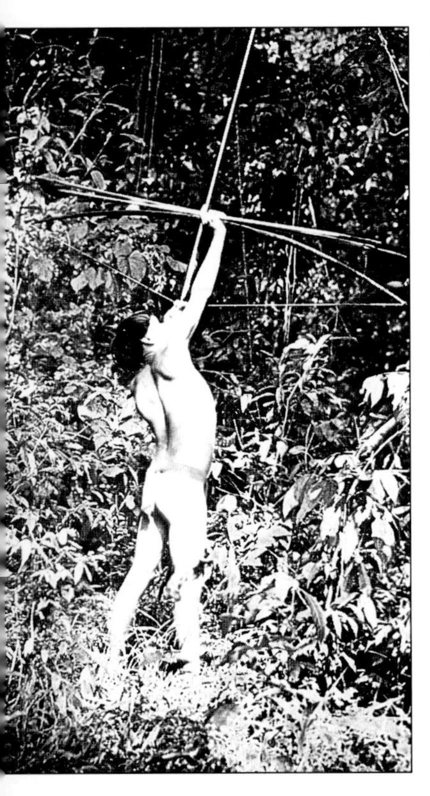

Indians are fascinated with weapons, but they still prefer their own traditional weaponry. Arrows are more useful for hunting because they are silent. An arrow won't scare a flock of birds as a gunshot would. In warfare, it's harder for an enemy to discern the origin of a silent arrow than that of a gunshot.

Before long we heard a gentle rumbling, then at the next bend in the river we saw the source: a waterfall, not too high, but very powerful nonetheless. Ian slowed down and made for the bank.

"I'm going to take a shortcut which will save us about a hundred kilometers. But we'll have to carry the boat for about two kilometers."

Seriously?

He looked at us as if to size us up. "Yeah, you're strong enough. You'll do."

Ian stayed in the boat while we took the supplies and the outboard motor ashore and carried them the two kilometers. Once at our destination, Norbert stayed behind to hide everything, and we went to get Ian's cargo, including the chicken cage. Then we carried the diesel tanks. Finally, all four of us returned and with Ian we hauled, dragged, pushed, and carried the boat which weighed a good three hundred kilograms. The hull was slippery as an eel, and the ropes we used to pull it cut into our skin from shoulder to hip as we dragged the boat over cliffs and stones.

When we had finished, Ian said, "Go get some firewood. We've earned our supper. But be careful, there are a lot of nasty spiders and snakes."

It was incredible. We were only about fifty paces from the sunny riverbed, and here it seemed as if we were in the darkest jungle, protected by a roof of leaves and branches. There was almost no undergrowth, and it was relatively easy to walk. But there was no firewood to be found. We'd have to go back to the riverbank to find some undergrowth and scrub, whether we wanted to or not.

As we returned to the camp, Ian had already started a modest fire. There was a scrawny bird on a spit, gutted and split. How did Ian do it? We didn't hear any shots, otherwise we would have come running to him right away. I looked at the cage. Three sad-looking chickens were mourning inside. "Our savior, the rooster!" I thought. He was one first-rate bird.

Four days later, Ian let us off at the Rio Demini.

"Well, our little excursion is over. The next stretch is impassable by boat. Stay near the river and you can't miss the Toototobi. It meets the Demini in three separate streams. That's how you'll recognize it."

I counted his money, and asked, "How will you make it back through the waterfall?"

"I won't. I'll take the long way around. Good luck."

The motor started up, and Ian was on his way.

That's the most he said to us during the entire trip. We never heard the long story about how he came from Holland, or how he lives in Moura on the Rio Negro, or how one can make a living by transporting rubber, or how one protects oneself from piranhas. But every year he still sends me a Christmas card.

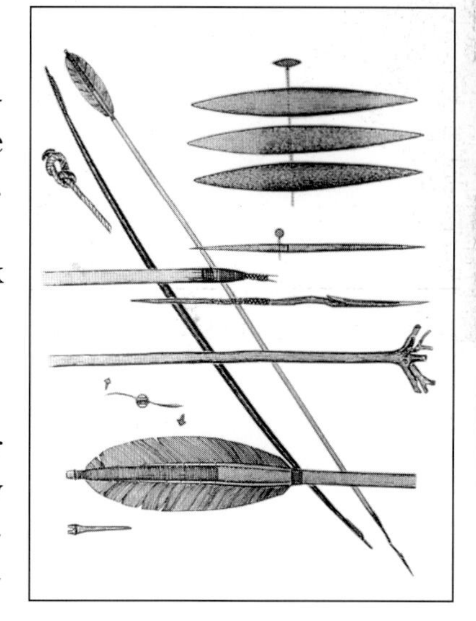

Although the Yanomamo never developed a written alphabet or number system, with only a glance they can notice a single arrow missing from among a bundle of twenty or thirty.

It's possible that he hadn't expected four bruisers like us, and maybe he was a little bit afraid of us. And I still laugh when I think about our first night in the rainforest, when we were terrified that Ian could actually do what he had said and make us disappear one after the other. As he had said himself, "Never trust the last white man you see before you go into the rainforest."

Peter had taken these words to heart as well. He had wandered away from our camp, and come across another human, probably a down-on-his-luck gold prospector. Peter was terrified, but, before he could say a word, the other had disappeared without a trace. After that, we decided to keep the night watch in pairs. Better safe than sorry.

The Wisdom of the Shamans

After seven days and countless smaller rivers (which we had become quite adept at crossing without falling in, just out of reach of the creatures for which we had developed a grudging respect), we came to a wider river. Our GPS device put us at 63°30´ longitude and 1°33´ latitude. We wound our way west, and sure enough, in four hours we came to a place where the river forked off toward the Demini. Two hours later, we came to another fork in the same direction.

According to Ian's description and our coordinates, this must be the Toototobi. Three Yanomamo warriors, who seemed to have appeared out of the blue, also confirmed this for us. Unlike Ian, or Peter's gold prospector, these three were quite chatty. Despite our weapons, they seemed to feel at ease on their home turf.

They appeared to be hunting. One proudly carried a gutted wild boar on his shoulder. The blood was still dripping. We gringos had looked in vain for such delicacies. Another had two wild chickens tucked into his belt. The third was carrying a bundle of about twenty bamboo rods under his arm. We explained, with great difficulty, that we were looking for a Maloka (village hut) which was the home of a young boy who had been treated by a white shaman in the city. I explained that I was the shaman from the city, and that I wanted to visit my young patient. They seemed to have heard of him. With the help of our Yanomamo-German phrase book, I repeated our questions several times, and each time they answered excitedly and gestured toward the west. Luckily, this was the direction we had expected.

I asked how many days travel we had ahead of us. One of the warriors made a sweeping motion from east to west: one sunrise, and one sunset, which is to say one day. They took us to a place where (in their opinion) we could safely cross the Demini. We gave them no gifts. Dieter had told me never to give any gifts to any warriors while they were out hunting. The body language on our departure, as they waved to us and we waved back, told me Dieter had been right.

More experienced now than we had been on our first day, we were able to cover three to four kilometers per hour, and to stay on the move from morning until night. We took a break of about one hour to orient ourselves and to give me time to make entries in my logbook, in which I entered any details I might have noticed, as if I were making notes of the cliffs and shoals of an unknown coastline in a nautical logbook.

In a patch of light, we could see a solitary mountain to the north. It rose from the earth like some great green wave. Could that be the place that had been marked "elevation unknown" on the map Dieter had given me, and which Peter had found so fascinating in the Café Landtmann? Now, he seemed to have absolutely no interest in finding out. His ear had become swollen and infected, and was quite painful. We had each taken something out of his backpack to lighten his load. I had advised him not to take any antibiotics. We would soon be arriving in the village, and he'd be able to rest for a while, and hopefully recover fairly quickly.

"Don't worry, I don't want any now. The shaman will be there, and maybe he'll give me some tea and make my body and soul healthy," said Peter. He was making an effort not to show us that he was in pain.

Norbert still had a fever. "But only at night," he said again and again, clenching his teeth.

What we had secretly feared came true. We took not one but three days to reach the village. A group of Indian scouts met us and took us to Katunka's (or Mauricio's) Maloka. I wondered how long they had been keeping an eye on us. First, we needed to rest for a few days. Norbert's condition had worsened. He started taking antibiotics, and we gathered rainwater, and gave him some tea every hour.

The village consisted of an artfully built structure made of bamboo and other sorts of vegetation, which formed a nearly perfect oval with a partial roof. It was similar to the oval shape of a bullfighting arena. The thatched roof was supported by perpendicular bamboo poles placed every four meters or so. Every pole marked the approximate limits of a separate living space. The walls which separated each space were made of thatched mats, which simply hung from the roof.

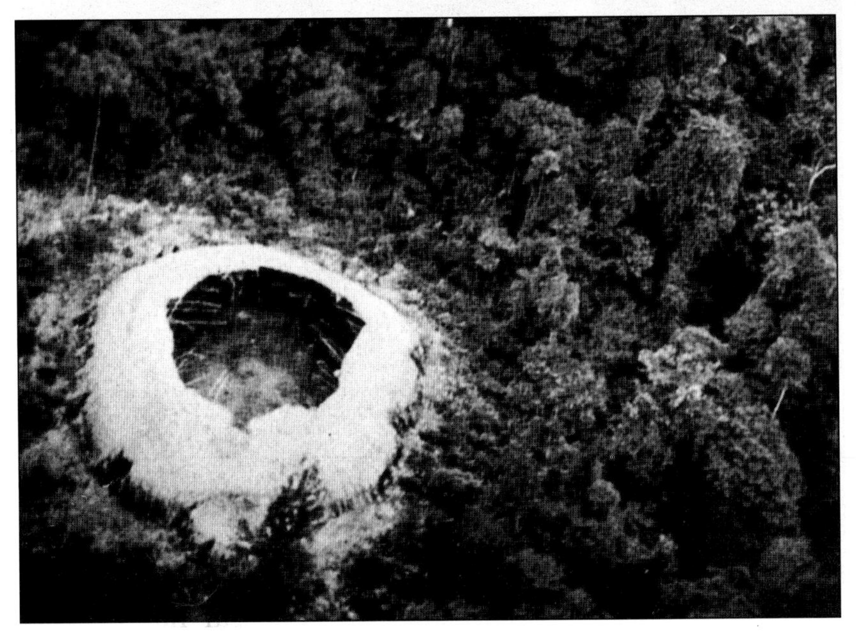

A Yanomamo Maloka from a bird's-eye view. Malokas are well suited to their surroundings. Population of the Maloka and the size of the oval never exceed a sustainable limit. The damage to the rainforest begins to heal a few months after the Indians have moved on.

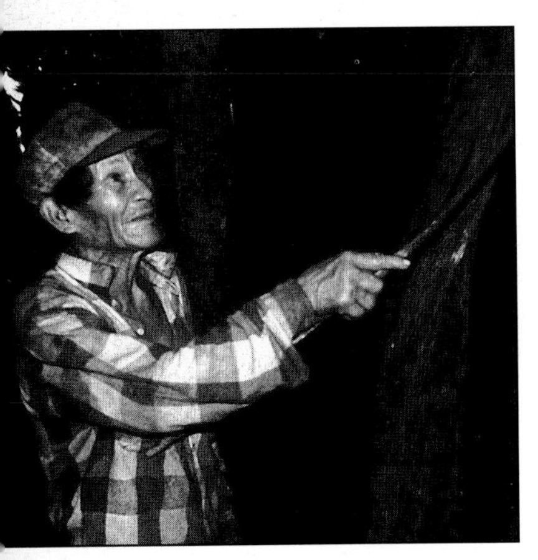

Blue jeans and war paint: the shaman, Katunka, wise and ready to learn, a blessing for his tribe.

The open space in the middle of the oval served as a play space for the children. They were forbidden to run into the forest alone. Nonetheless, we later observed that some of them, always the same ones, felt some kind of magical attraction to the forest. This reminded me of city children who are compelled to play in the streets or in strange neighborhoods, despite protests from their parents. I thought that, with the exception of a few aluminum pots, this village looked just as one might have looked thirty thousand years ago. The difference was that there were many more Yanomamo thirty thousand years ago than there are today. Some researchers claim that there were as many as three million Indians in this region before the arrival of the white man. As recently as the 1960s it was not uncommon for whites to go hunting for Indians, just as white settlers in Australia used to go hunting for aborigines.

When we arrived in the Maloka on the third day, Katunka (I'm going to stick with this name) approached us with his characteristic erect bearing, just as he had in the hospital in Sao Paulo. Instead of jeans, he wore only a tiny belt and was otherwise naked. There were smallish women standing around, quite plump and stark naked. They had plucked their pubic hairs, which seemed to accentuate their nakedness. The children were so busy playing that they hardly noticed us.

I could see only a few men. Gradually, more men began to appear, keeping a respectful distance behind Katunka. Katunka lifted his hands in a gesture of welcome, and then

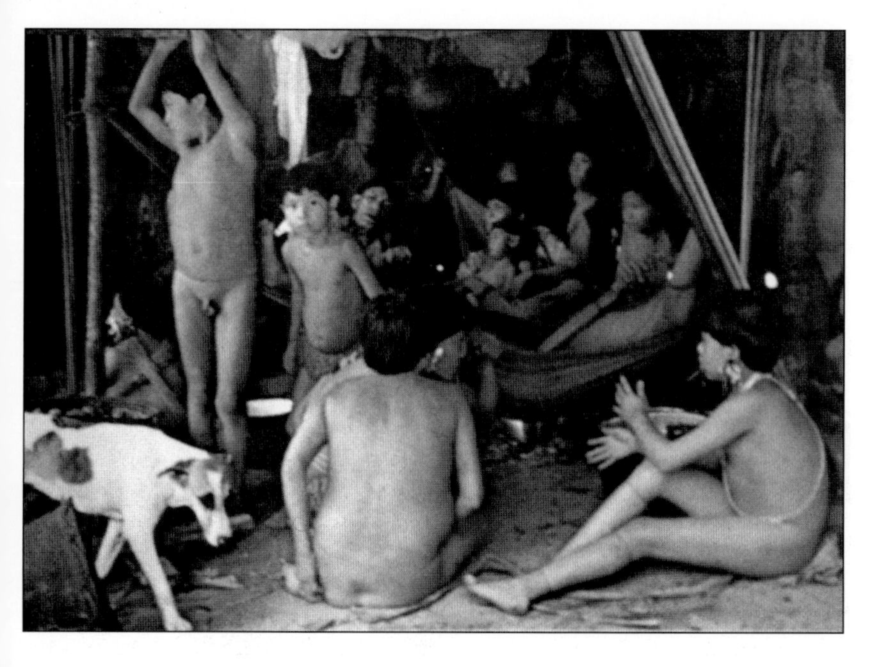

Cleanliness and hygiene are of primary importance in the Maloka. Even the dogs are kept scrupulously clean. The ubiquitous "jungle outhouse" also helps to maintain sanitary conditions. Countless insects and microbes work to break down feces so efficiently that it disappears without a trace within a few hours.

began a welcoming oration of which we understood only the final two words in Portuguese: "Bom dia" (Good day).

Everything was going as planned. It had taken us thirteen days to come here from Manaus. How long we would be able to stay depended on our return trip. Katunka was of inestimable help, as he would be so often during our stay. He had arranged for warriors from a friendly neighboring tribe to take us by canoe on the Demini to Ramao, which, according to the map, we had passed with Ian but hadn't seen. From there, we would take the "tuktuktuk" to Marova where we would take the *Emerson Madeiros* back to Manaus.

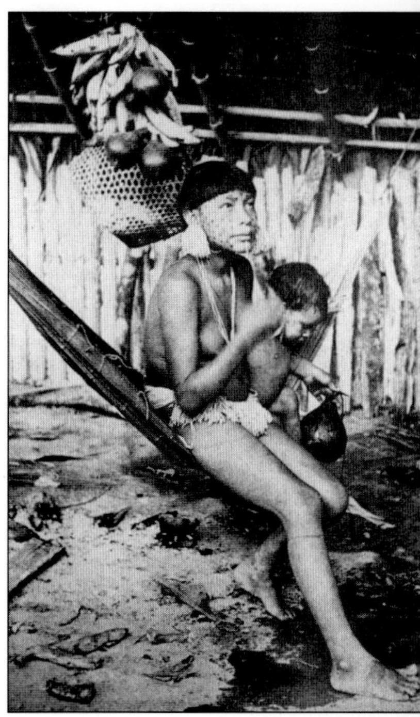

It was two days before all this was explained to us, but we would still be able to stay two full weeks. Considering all the planning and preparation I had done for this trip, I assumed that the Indians would have a difficult time understanding our relative haste. But to the wise old man, it seemed, for whatever reason, child's play.

Now it became imperative for us to begin to understand our hosts. When would the right moment arrive to bring up the subject of the plants? And then there was (I almost wrote "luckily!") Peter's infected ear, which I showed to Katunka after our arrival. His gestures said, "Yes, it must hurt, but it'll go away eventually."

I wasn't so certain, however, and said to Peter, "Go ahead and take some antibiotics. It doesn't make any sense for you to suffer."

On the third day, the young boy on whom Dieter had operated in Sao Paulo suddenly appeared. I wanted to ask him where he had been hiding.

He reached out to shake my hand, and spoke to me in Portuguese which was much better than my own. Incredibly, our young patient had picked up the language while he was in the hospital in Sao Paulo.

I gave him a couple of peppermint candies and he was beside himself. I asked him his name, and he answered like a gunshot, "Thomas." I had secretly hoped to become friends with him, but I was to be sorely disappointed.

It was Freddy's fault. Freddy and his kazoo. He had made a kazoo out of a comb and a chewing gum wrapper, and all the children in the village followed him everywhere he went. Once Thomas had finished all the peppermint candies I gave him, he seemed more interested in that kazoo than in anything else in the world. This was the only musical instrument on which Freddy had even a marginal mastery, so he was not eager to part with it.

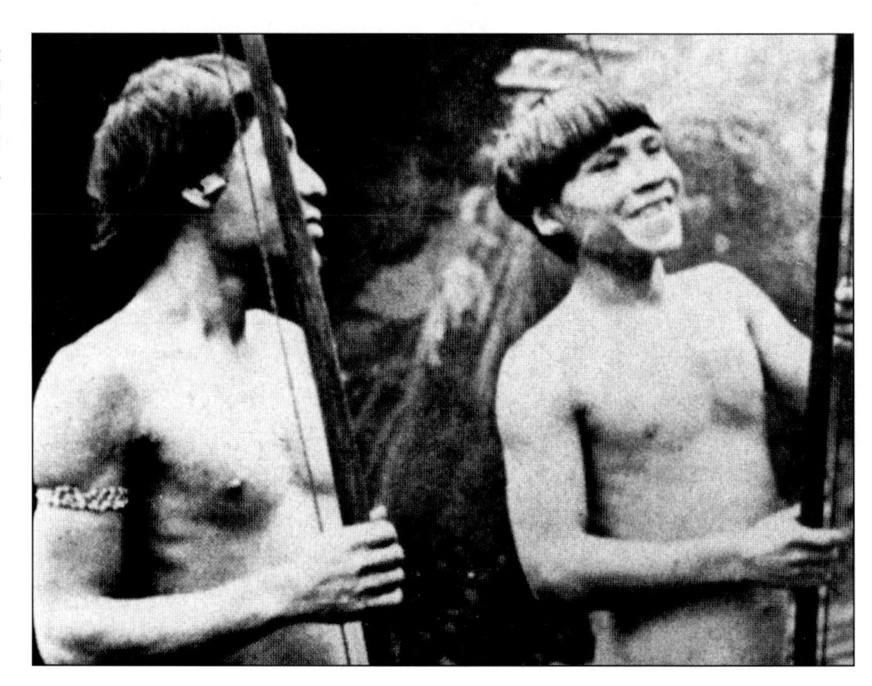

A simple twist of fate: A hip operation on Suma, a young Indian boy *(right)*, led me to the Yanomamo and CoD Tea.

Up to that point, I had been downright miserly in handing out presents. I didn't want to give the impression that I had come to buy their friendship and their botanical knowledge. Before I tried such methods, I wanted to learn as much as pos-

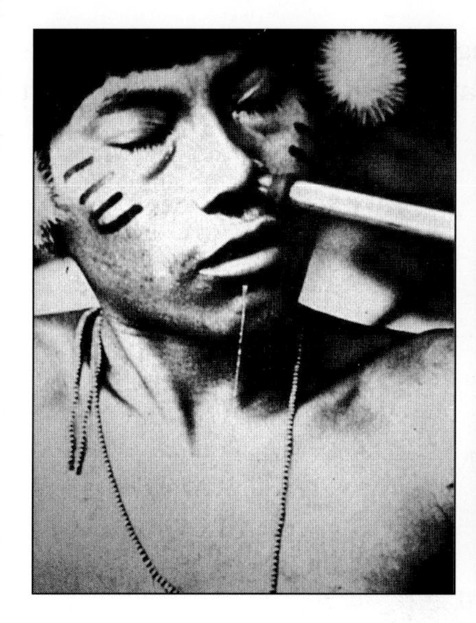
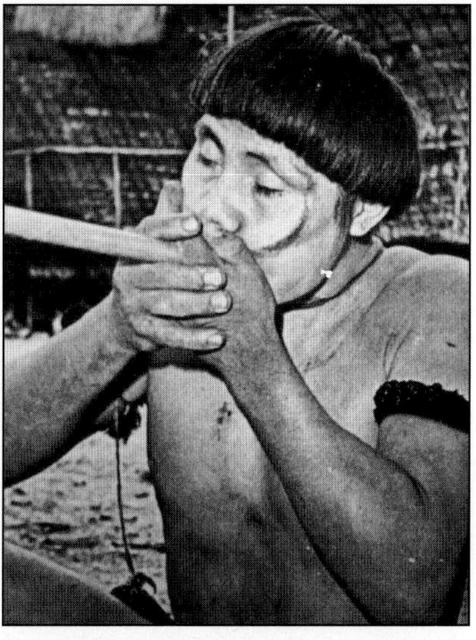

Before a ritual celebration, the Yanomamo get themselves "high" by blowing a powerful drug into one another's noses.

sible about their way of thinking and their reactions to various situations, and, in the worst case, go home with some unfinished business, with plans to return in a year.

We had already decided that we each wanted to spend at least a couple of hours on our own alone each day, which would allow us each the opportunity to make friends separately.

Lying in our hammocks at night, we'd compare notes on how we were doing. When I thumb through my journal today, I find it filled with entries such as the following:

"Today Freddy and some children helped some women working in the gardens. They were growing manioc (which is used to make flour for a special kind of pocket bread that they use), some tobacco, cotton, and bananas. This can't possibly be enough to feed the entire tribe. The women are very capable, but the ground is uncooperative, and the topsoil is very thin."

In another entry, I noted, "Norbert has counted 72 women, 46 children, and only 18 adult males, including Katunka. Even if you figure an average of two women for every man, that means some are missing. Where are they? Out hunting? Peter says that he feels he's being watched all the time, especially when he steps out to 'take care of his business.' Freddy is convinced that a young woman is making eyes at him (trying to flirt with him). She has been seen with some rowdy young boys that he's been hanging out with."

Katunka spent some time with us every morning and evening, but on the fifth day, he had disappeared. Slowly, we were starting to become bored.

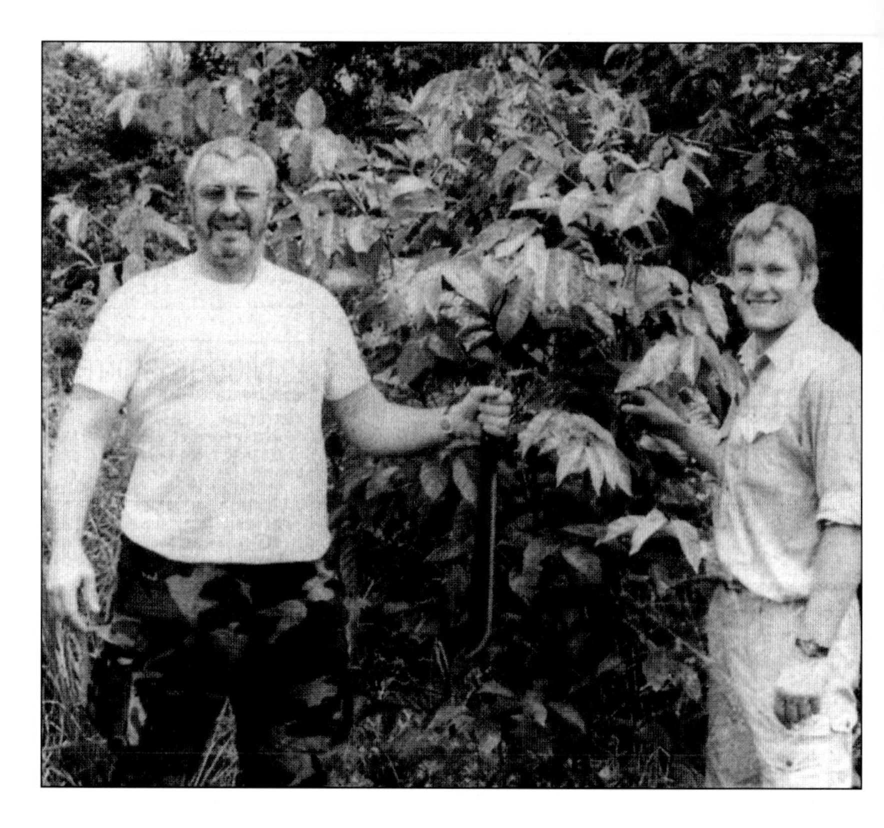

Hunting for medicinal plants with Peter Seisenbacher. Actually, the picture is somewhat misleading. In reality we always had a native with us to keep us from getting lost. It takes only a few steps in the jungle for an inexperienced hiker to lose his or her way.

The many travel writers whose books I had read had nothing on us. In just a few days we had seen a celebration of death in which a corpse was put in a net and hung from a tree (which is actually a widespread custom); women from a neighboring tribe were kidnapped, which led to some hair-raising skirmishes; we saw wild spiritual rituals celebrated under the influence of mind-altering drugs; and babies came into the world. But for Freddy the high point was a native woman flirting with him and I was not amused.

The Maloka Treaty

On the seventh day, everything had changed. About twenty warriors suddenly stood around the walls of the village. Katunka was with them. I did not recognize him at first; his body was painted.

"Oh boy, now it's getting serious," said Freddy.

The women greeted the men in a less-than-cheerful manner.

"No wonder," I thought, "they haven't brought anything home for dinner."

Katunka came toward us with a large man who seemed to be a chief of some sort, and another man I had not seen before.

Their movements were wooden and stiff. The one I hadn't seen before was the translator. He stepped to the front, greeted us in Portuguese, and began to describe the situation at hand.

According to the translator, it seems that, a few days on foot from here, on the "Perimetral Norte" road, there was a conflict. All manner of riffraff and unsavory characters made the areas near the road unsafe, much as they still do today. They say about the gold prospectors that "if they have no luck prospecting, maybe they'll be lucky enough to run into you." What this meant was that they had no qualms about robbing (or murdering) an innocent person if their luck was running out.

The interpreter continued to report that the gringos had fought with some Indians, and men from both sides had been killed. It was possible that the gringos would show up here, near the village. Then he asked if we wanted to leave.

Peter took a step toward the chief, added at least an inch to his height by standing as upright as possible, and said, "Maybe if we stay, the gringos will go away."

The interpreter translated. Soon everything grew silent, even the constant rustling of the trees around the village clearing. Then the chief handed his arrow over to the interpreter, came to us, and shook hands European style. Freddy said to us in German, "I hope you realize that what we're doing is most definitely not in the spirit of Austrian neutrality."

This handshake sealed what we called the "Malokan Peace and Friendship Treaty." From that point on the Indians rewarded us with their unconditional trust and Alton, the interpreter, stood by us and was always close at hand.

The first thing I learned from Alton was less than flattering. The Indians had not seen us as a source of protection, in spite of our weapons, our strength, and our size. We were too clumsy with our weapons, laughed Alton.

Katunka was counting on our help, not as fighters but merely for our presence as whites. In this respect, he acted much as former Austrian Chancellor Bruno Kreisky had. At one time, Austria was planning to invest in a multibillion-dollar U.N. site in Vienna. Naturally, the plan came under heavy criticism, which he responded to by saying, "This investment will bring more to the security of our country than one thousand new tanks. No one would possibly care to face the diplomatic consequences of occupying a country which was home to the United Nations."

According to Alton, the strategy of the Indians was similar.

"Katunka said that if garimpeiros come to take revenge, they might think that these whites (here he gestured toward us) are officers from FUNAI. The garimpeiros will not kill, but will leave for fear that the whites will lock them up."

Peter had spoken to the chief directly from his heart and soul, and he had said exactly what the chief had wanted to hear.

"What makes you think we're so clumsy?" asked Norbert, somewhat insulted.

Alton explained that his tribe had posted spies everywhere to keep a lookout for garimpeiros. They had been watching us all the way from the river. Then he imitated our stumbling and tripping, stopping to wipe off the sweat, fanning ourselves with our hats, and—smacking hear and there—he imitated us slapping ourselves in a futile attempt to relieve the constant torment of mosquitoes.

The landmark botanical text *Historia Naturalis Palmarum*, from the early nineteenth century, was filled with true-to-life illustrations. For the first time, color lithographs revealed in exquisite detail the flowers and fruits of tropical palms.

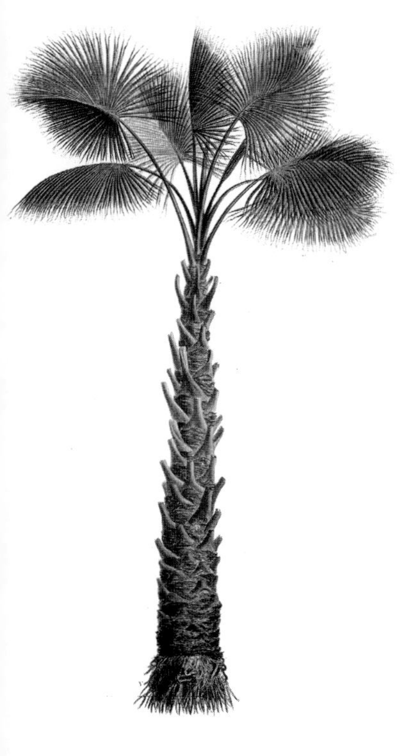

"And how did you know that we weren't garimpeiros?"

"Garimpeiros no click machine, no red cross, no pens."

Alton, who was not such a stranger to the outside world as he might seem, had recognized our camera, the red cross on my medicine bag, and my stopping to make constant notations on my map. It is likely that this paraphernalia had saved our lives. That also explains why the three warriors we met in the forest were so open and trusting.

I suddenly wondered aloud, "Oh God, we should tell Alton about the white man that Peter met so he can warn the chief."

"He's dead," said Alton.

It seemed a good time to ask questions, so I asked about young Thomas. "How did Thomas end up having surgery in the city of the whites?"

"Who?"

I told him about the hip operation in Sao Paulo.

"Oh, Suma. He was at the FUNAI hospital on the Demini with Katunka. They took him to the city."

FUNAI operates several clinics in the Indian regions of the Amazon. A doctor who had determined that the boy needed an operation knew about our new technique. Later we also learned that Katunka had been acquainted with the Villa Lobos brothers (the founders of FUNAI) and was often invited to represent his people at official government conferences.

That explained a lot. I had asked myself at least a hundred times how a young Indian boy from a tiny village in the middle of the rainforest ends up at the University Clinic in Sao Paulo to be operated on for a condition which is not exactly life threatening. And, given the distance, how is it possible that a relative comes to visit, as if he only had to hop on the local bus?

"Is Katunka your shaman?" I asked.

"Katunka wise man, shaman, father of Chief Shururi. Chief Shururi shaman, too."

"I am a shaman of the whites. I would like to learn from Katunka. Katunka is a wise man, and many years old. I am still young. He can teach me much," I said.

"Tomorrow," said Alton.

That night, all the men gathered by the fire. Katunka and Chief Shururi just chewed their tobacco, and neither said much.

Norbert, the only smoker in our group, offered Shururi a cigarette. The chief took the entire pack, quickly ripped open a cigarette, tucked the paper neatly in his belt, and made a ball with the moist tobacco. He put this in his mouth and began to chew. He seemed to be relishing the experience.

"Well, there were only nine left," said Norbert, somewhat down in the mouth from losing his stash. He didn't know that I had two whole cartons of the repulsive poison in my backpack. His birthday was in two days, and I wanted to celebrate by surprising him with them.

Norbert made such a long face that I was tempted not to wait until his birthday.

With the Blessings of the Spirits

Early the next morning Alton came to us, and said, "School."

It came as no surprise that he knew the word. The previous day he had told me that FUNAI had established several Indian schools further up on the Demini. On a later trip on the Rio Madeira we visited one of these schools. Children within a radius of twenty miles were transported by boat to their lessons. The school also had a clinic, a red cross station, and a hospital for local natives. Everything was spotless and well equipped.

Alton stood and waited impatiently like a school bus driver in the American midwest, until I had packed my paraphernalia. We crossed the center of the Maloka to a place where Katunka stood waiting for us. Alton left with a wave of Katunka's hand.

Katunka had prepared himself like an experienced schoolmaster.

I had noticed that he placed great regard on formality and ceremony. He was wearing the same jeans he had worn in the hospital in Sao Paulo. Lacking a demonstration table, various plants and pieces of tree bark sat neatly ordered on the ground. Add an ink jar, blackboard, and chalk and we would have had a perfect classroom.

Just as my teachers from my Hungarian childhood used to do, Katunka signaled for to me to sit down. More than likely he had learned the gesture at the FUNAI school on the river. I guessed that he had also attended various conferences and lectures in the cities, and had probably given some talks himself. Alton had already implied as much, and later this would be confirmed.

I crouched on the ground. Everything was dead quiet for a second. Then my teacher began to babble incomprehensibly. I looked at him in exasperation, but his eyes were closed. After a short time, he said to me in Portuguese, "I have asked the great spirits that they should bless what we are doing here. All will be well with my tribe, with all the Indians of the rivers and forests, and the whites under the morning sun. Now you speak to the great spirit of the whites, and we can begin the lesson."

He wanted me to pray.

My God! I was prepared for almost anything but that. It was morning, but I could only think of a bedtime prayer that my grandmother taught me when I was just a child. So I began hesitantly, *"Dear God, do not forsake us in the evening of the day, in the evening of our life, and do us honor on judgment day."*

The old man looked at me expectantly. Had I done something wrong? Had I forgotten something?

I said "Amen."

"Amen," he repeated. Satisfied, he began his presentation.

Everything Katunka had learned about his people and the power of the forest, about the animals on the land and the fish in the water and the birds in the air, he had learned from his father. His father was a great shaman who had the power to wake the dead. This is why he was kidnapped by another tribe. "We never saw him again," said Katunka.

His family had searched for him to the point of exhaustion. Even then I had a vague idea of how terrible the kidnapping must have been for Katunka. He and his family were in agony wondering whether his father's soul would go to heaven. There are two factors which determine this. First, the body is bound in a net and hung from a tree until ants and other insects leave only the bones, which are then burned and eaten by the survivors of the deceased. Then the soul must pass a test upon arriving in the hereafter.

This must at least partially explain why even today tribes are really nothing more than extended families. Who else would eat the ashes of a dead acquaintance?

There are also tribes who bury their dead. And if the tribe should move on for any reason, the bones of the deceased are dug up and taken along to the new village.

Katunka also described quite clearly the misfortunes of the Indians since the arrival of the whites:

"Everything the whites bring is good and bad. The gun good. *Boom*, garimpeiro dead. But other garimpeiros hear boom and come to kill. Gun good. *Boom*, and animal dead. But other animals hear boom, and run away. Indian arrow only good, not bad. *Ffft*, garimpeiro dead. *Ffft*, animal dead. *Ffft*, more animals dead."

Should I have interjected here that the war of the whites is so loud that the crack of a rifle is drowned out in the din of a battle? And that when a hunter shoots a deer, he probably won't eat it, but will hang its head on the wall of his Maloka? It would have only narrowed, and not increased his understanding of white culture, so I let it go. Besides, as the student, it wasn't my place to interrupt my teacher.

I gathered from the rest of his talk that he thought there were only two kinds of whites. One (the good white? successful? rich?) stayed at home in their cities. The other (the bad white? unsuccessful? a loser? incompetent?) came to the rainforest to live and to drive away the Indians. The same principle applies when a tribe packs up and moves on when an area can no longer provide sustenance; it destroys any tribe that stands in its way.

It's still the same today, not just because of the white prospectors exploring for gold, but because of the many tribal wars. I'd like to quote Tom Sterling, a Briton who has concerned himself with this theme for the Food and Agriculture Organization of the United Nations. He writes, "Most Europeans who must live here without supplies from the outside will soon run the risk of starving to death. But the Indians get by without supplies from the outside, and still they survive. How is it possible? The answer to this puzzle is found in the astounding and often dismaying information regarding how humans must behave in order to live in harmony with Nature. One of the first and most disturbing results of the shortage of food supply is that the few groups of Indians in the Amazon region have a tendency toward violence. A shortage of food means that a limited amount of resources must be divided up among the various tribes. If these tribes, which are little more than extended families, have to roam in search of food, eventually they will encroach on another tribe's terrain."

Despite his understanding, even a man having as much wisdom and experience as Katunka was convinced that the only whites who had bothered to settle in the rainforest were those who had been cast out or for whom there was a shortage of food. Perhaps the human refuse of the slums of South American cities had done something to convince him of this.

We were fortunate. What distinguished us from the other whites who had trekked deep into the jungle was that we were invited.

Before I go on with the details of my first lesson, I'd like to quote Tom Sterling again, in order to illustrate how critical we must be when reading reports on the rainforest and its inhabitants. Sterling continued the quote I mentioned above, as follows:

"The assertions of romantically disposed outsiders that all Indians live together in perfect harmony with themselves and Nature and consider only whites to be the enemy is utter nonsense. The most dangerous enemies the Indian has are other Indians.

"Many observers hold the view that the Indian system of war and violence is a method of population control, insuring that the demand for food does not exceed the limited supply. The number of murderous *Jivaros* remains stable. There is approximately one person per every three square kilometers of land, and we can conclude that that is exactly what the land can support. In the last fifteen thousand years, the Amazon has probably never seen more than a total native population of 3,000,000."

Today, however, there are only 200,000 to 300,000. Personally, I cannot agree with the statement that the Indians' most dangerous enemies are other Indians, when the whites have been carrying out an unacknowledged genocide, reducing the number of Indians from a high of 3,000,000 to a low of 200,000 or 300,000.

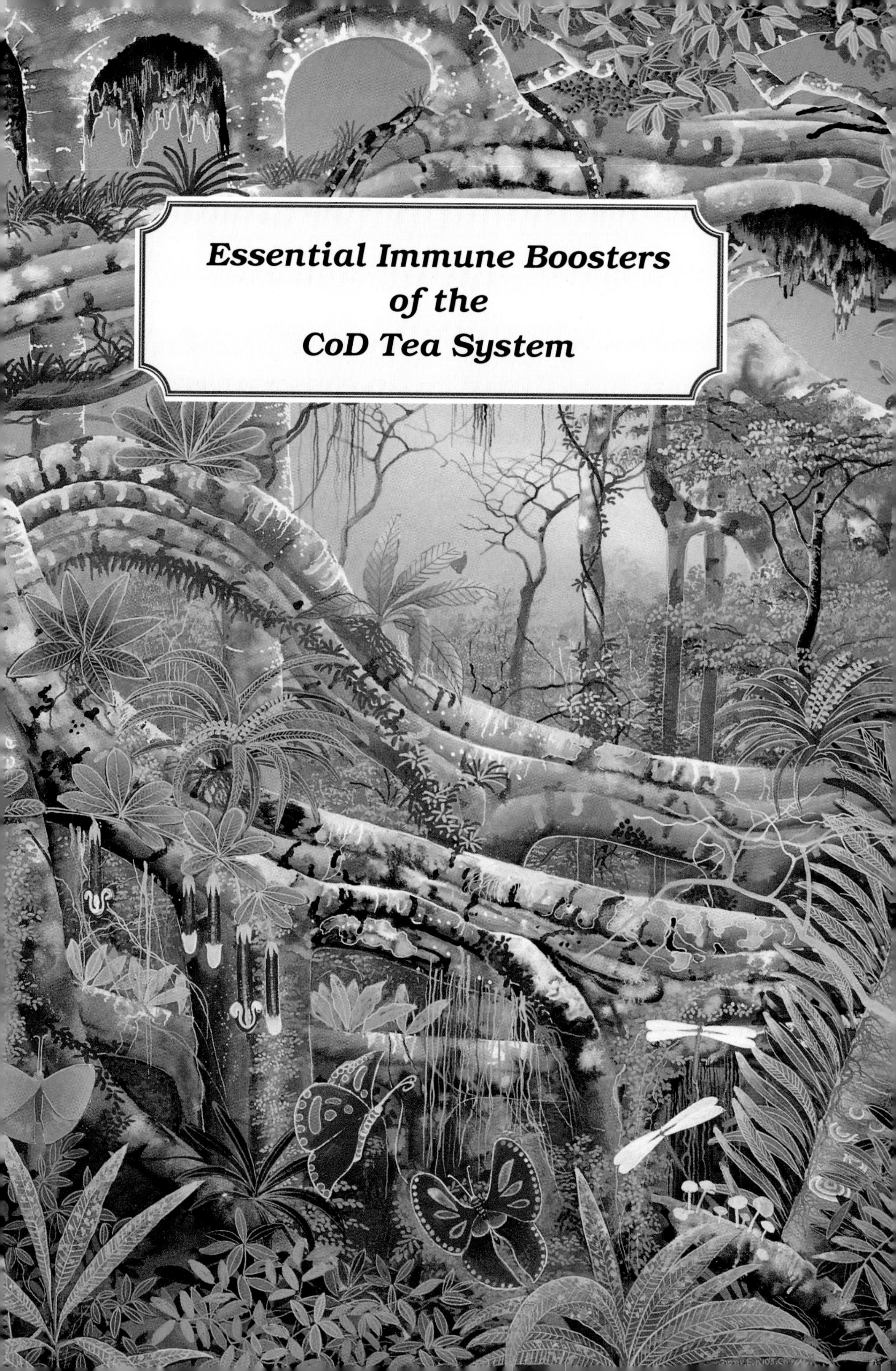
Essential Immune Boosters
of the
CoD Tea System

From the Shamans' Medicine Chest

The experience and practice of herbal medicine of the rainforest Indians shows that the attempts of native cultures to use plants for medicinal purposes is a universal phenomenon. It may surprise you to know that the Indians do have what we in the West normally think of as "modern" illnesses, those normally associated with Western industrial civilization. Take rheumatism, hemorrhoids, and gout, for example. Indians treat them with the same plants or plant extracts that we do in the West—in so far as they are locally available to them—and they also value such plants as garlic and nettles for the same reasons we do.

While the Indians have learned to harness the concentrated power of rainforest plants, Western researchers have only recently discovered what natives have known for millennia: the power of the largest forest on the planet lies not in the ground but in the plants themselves. If an area is damaged from a fire, the ashes will fertilize the soil to bring one or two generations of growth, and then it's all over.

A truly comprehensive botanical lexicon of rainforest plants has yet to be made. Pharmaceutical companies still pay rewards for samples of as-yet-undiscovered plants from this, the most diverse botanical area in the world. The plants illustrated in this book have been selected on the basis of their importance as ingredients of CoD Tea.

AGRIMONY, STICKLEWORT

Agrimonia eupatoria
Family: Rosaceae

This plant grows to a height of approximately 90 centimeters. It has numerous small, yellow flowers, and is found along riverbanks in the Amazon regions.

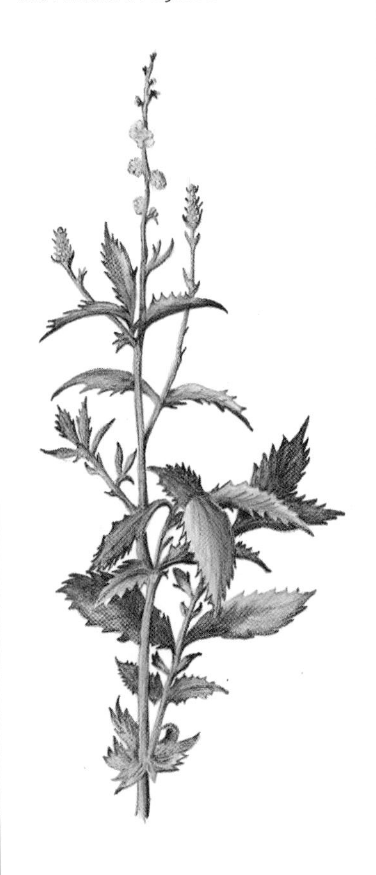

Used to treat: Liver deficiencies, diarrhea and abdominal cramps, kidney and bladder infections, asthma, inflammation of the throat, intestinal infections, digestive complications, typhus, and tumors. Used primarily as a diuretic and astringent.

A tea is brewed from the leaves and flowers. Also applied externally with compresses, and used as a mouthwash.

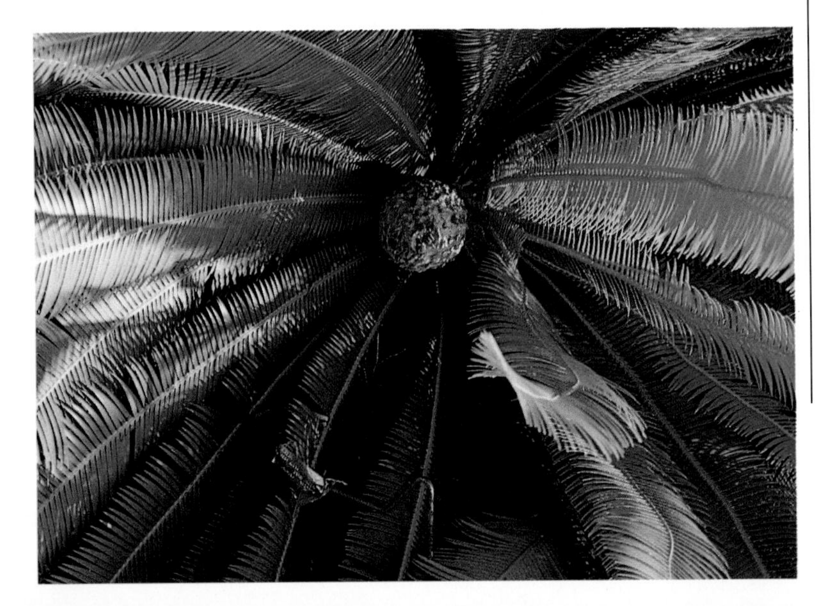

Roof, inner wall and outer wall. Palm trees provide Indians with building material, while the fruit serves as a sign of hospitality.

ANGELICA

Angelica archangelica
Family: Umbeliferaceae

Found near the rivers of the Amazon, it has white flowers and grows to a height of up to 2 meters.

Used to treat: Stomach and digestive problems, liver disfunction,

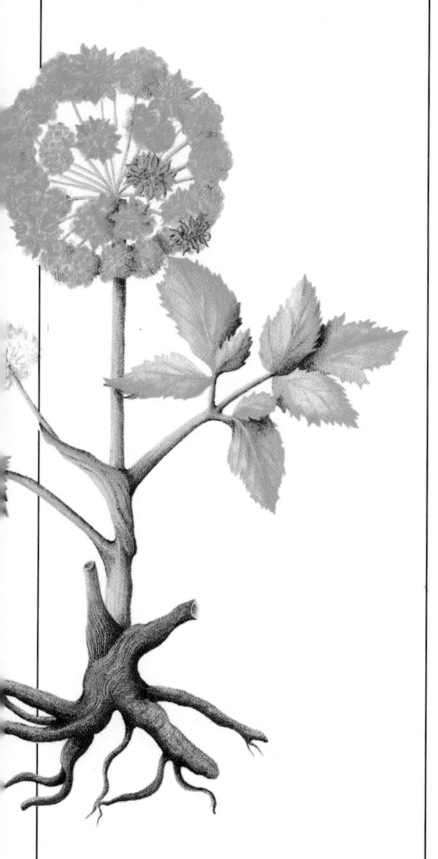

colic, bronchitis, tonsillitis, scurvy, gout, hysteria, rheumatism, tetanus, typhus, and menstrual complications.

The fruit, leaves, seeds, and roots can be used. Leaves and flowers can be used to make an infusion, and the fruit, seeds, and roots can be used in a decoction.

MUGWORT

Artemisia vulgaris
Family: Compositae

Found all over the Amazon region.

Used to treat: Anemia, colic, disruptions of the stomach, diarrhea, intestinal infections, epilepsy, jaundice, and worms.

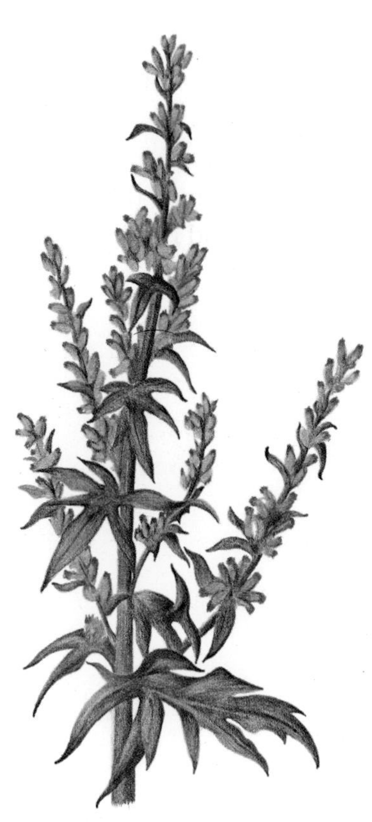

The entire plant can be used. Prepare an infusion of flowers and leaves for internal use. The roots can be cooked in boiling water for 15 minutes to make a decoction.

BEARBERRY

Arctostaphylos uvae ursi
Family: Ericaceae

Found near the rivers of the Amazon.

Used to treat: Bladder conditions, cystitis, kidney stones, and painful urination. It is used for its

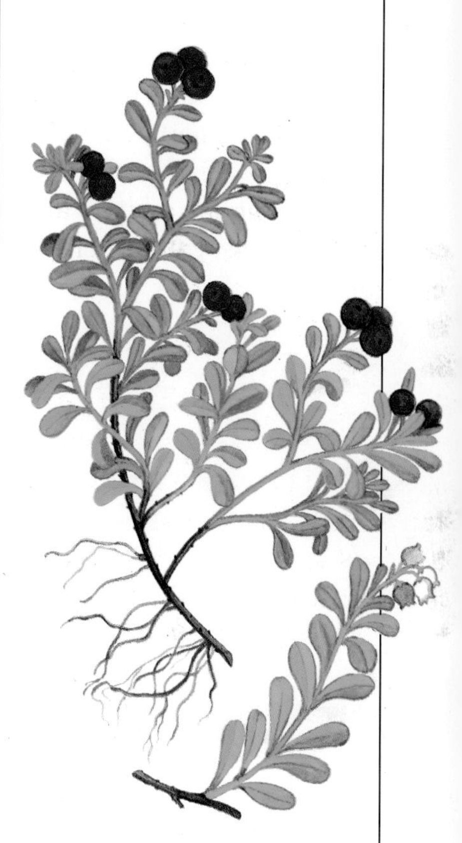

antiseptic qualities, and can help break up calculus in the urinary bladder, kidney stones, and gallstones.

Boil the leaves for 10 minutes to make a decoction.

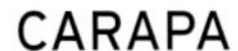

SHEPHERD'S PURSE

Capsella bursa pastoris
Family: Cruciferaceae

This plant has white flowers and grows to a height of approximately 60 centimeters. It is found throughout the Amazon.

Used to treat: Blood poisoning, vomiting, nosebleeds, bleeding of the uterus, and various tumors.

It is valued for its vasoconstrictor and styptic properties.

CARAPA

Carapa guianensis
Family: Meliaceae

An enormous tree which grows throughout the Amazon.

Used to treat: Worms and fever. It can also can be used externally for chronic inflammation of the

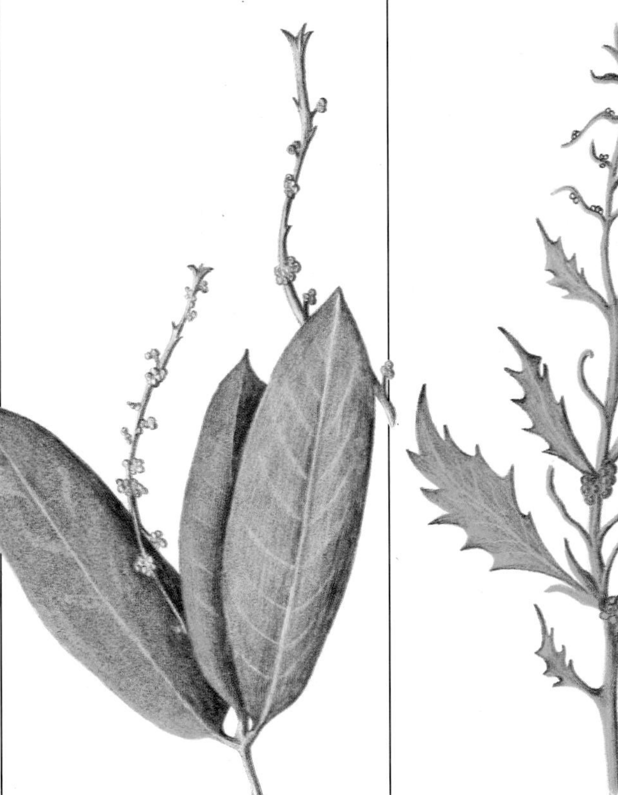

skin and as a detoxifier and purifier.

An extract made with alcohol works as an insect repellent.

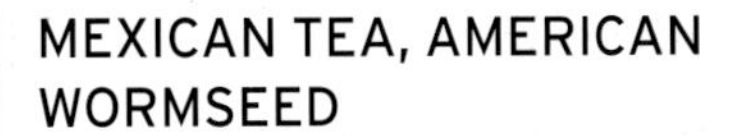

MEXICAN TEA, AMERICAN WORMSEED

Chenopodium ambrosioides
Family: Quenopodiaceae

Found throughout the Amazon.

Used as an insecticide, and against tuberculosis and worms. Can also be used externally in compresses, and as a mouthwash.

Tea can be made with an infusion. Use 20 grams of leaves for every liter of water. Take 3 cups a day.

Caution: Excessive doses can be harmful.

LICORICE

Glycyrrhiza glabra
Family: Leguminosae

A small tree which grows up to 2 meters. Grows along riverbanks in the Amazon.

Roots used to treat: Bronchitis, tonsillitis, and laryngitis.

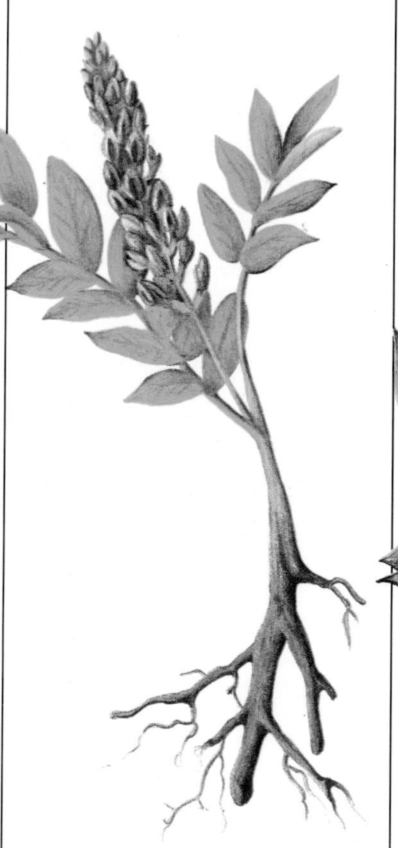

Use 20 grams of roots per liter of water to make a decoction. Take up to 5 cups a day.

JATOBA

Hymenaea courbaril
Family: Leguminosae

Found throughout the Amazon region.

Used to treat: Acute cystitis, prostatitis, excess or insufficient urine, and bronchitis. Helps relieve

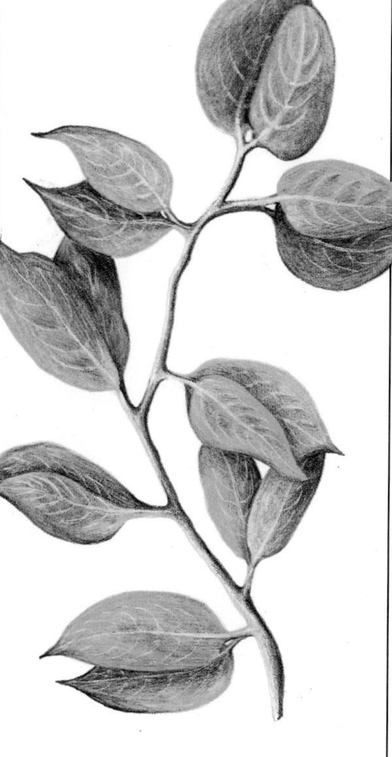

prostate conditions and swollen and painful joints.

Make a decoction from the bark, and drink with a little honey.

The sap is used to treat worms and stomach conditions, and as an astringent.

BLIND NETTLE

Lamium album
Family: Labiceae

This plant grows from 20 to 40 centimeters high and can be found throughout the Amazon.

Used to treat: Bleeding, festering wounds, menstrual difficulties,

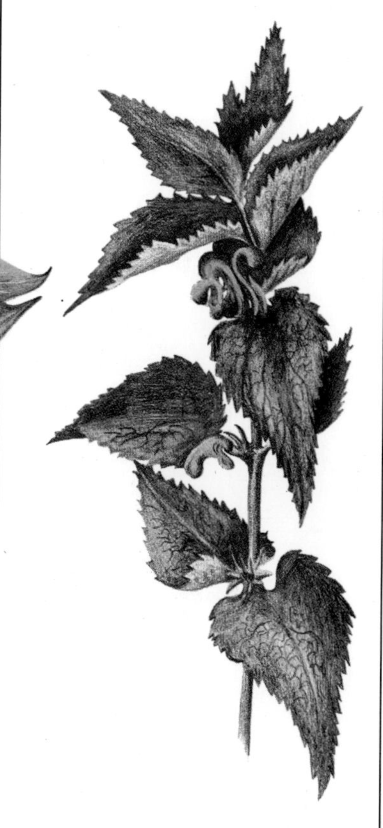

and inflamed ovaries. A wonderful treatment for all kinds of inflammation and catarrh of the air passages.

An infusion can be made from the leaves.

COMMON PLANTAIN

Plantago major
Family: Plantagenaceae

Found throughout the Amazon.

Used to treat: Anemia, gastritis, diarrhea, nephritis, cystitis, bleeding, pneumonia, tumors, and allergic reactions to insect bites.

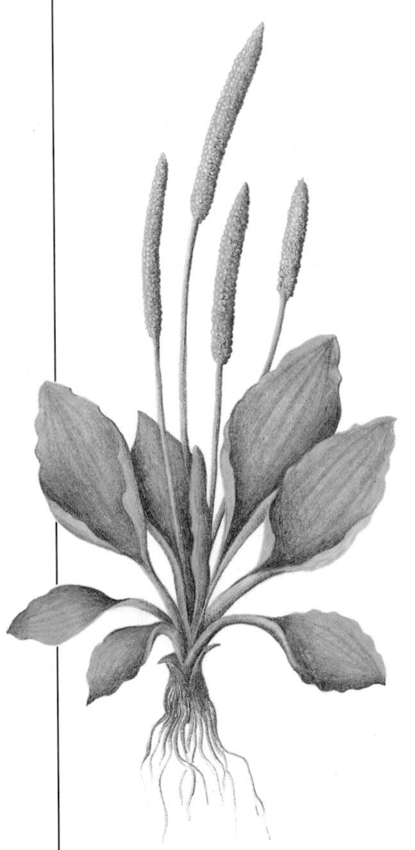

Both the leaves and the roots can be used. Make an infusion from the leaves, and a decoction from the roots. Make a compress to treat inflammation and infections of the eye while simultaneously drinking the infusion.

BASIL

Ocimum basilicum
Family: Labiacaeae

Found throughout the Amazon.

Used to treat: Calcium shortage due to childbirth; tonsillitis; intestinal conditions. Strengthens the bladder, and helps ease digestive discomfort.

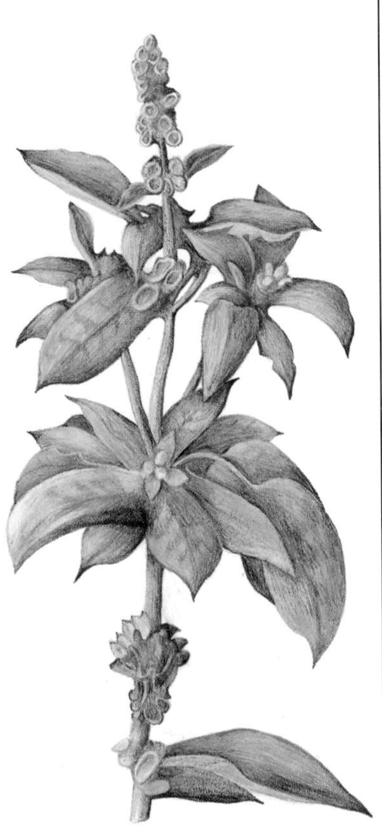

Make a tea from the leaves and the fresh flowers. In some areas, basil is also used to treat tuberculosis.

BRAZILIAN SASSAFRAS

Laurus sassafras
Family: Lauraceae

A tree that grows up to 12 meters high. Found in rainforests all over South America.

Used to treat: Dermatitis, arthritis, and gout. Also used to treat cases of metal poisoning and syphilis and to regulate perspiration.

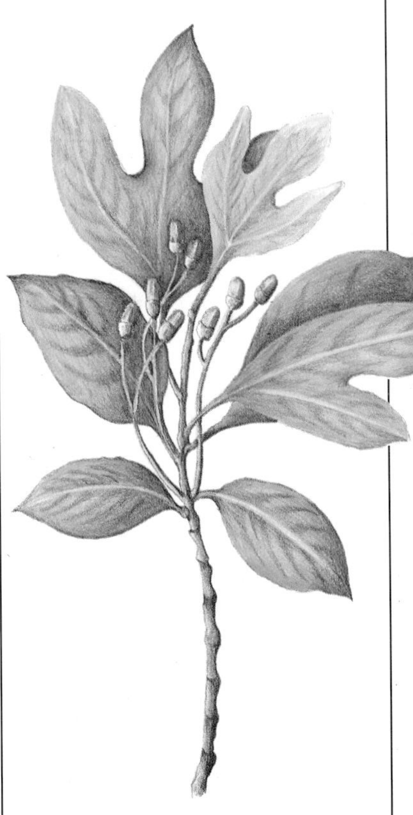

Make a decoction from the roots and the branches. Add 20 grams to 1 liter of water. Take up to 5 cups daily. Boil for 20 minutes.

PAU AMAGO

Quassia amara
Family: Simarubaceae

A small tree which is found throughout the Amazon.

Used to treat: Gallstones, kidney stones, stomach discomfort, diarrhea, and fever.

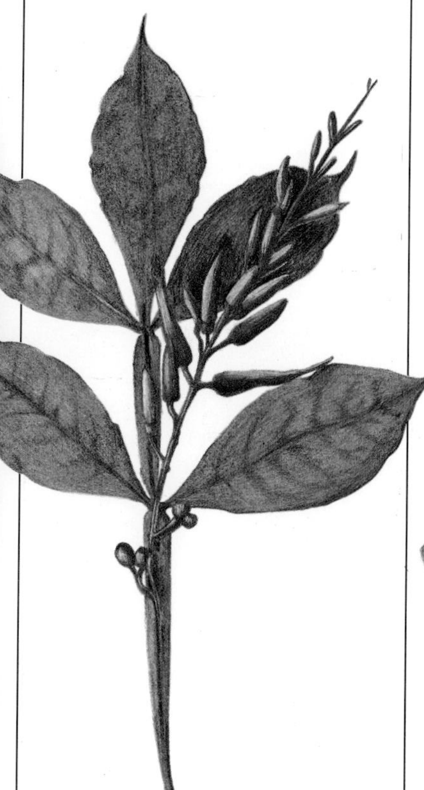

Make a tea from the bark and roots. Take up to 3 cups daily.

BOLDO

Peumus boldus molina
Family: Monimiaceae

Native to the riverbanks of the Amazon region.

Used to treat: Liver inflammation, liver disfunction, digestive problems, loss of appetite, gallstones, and gall colic. Enhances the effects of other medications used to treat bronchitis and tonsillitis.

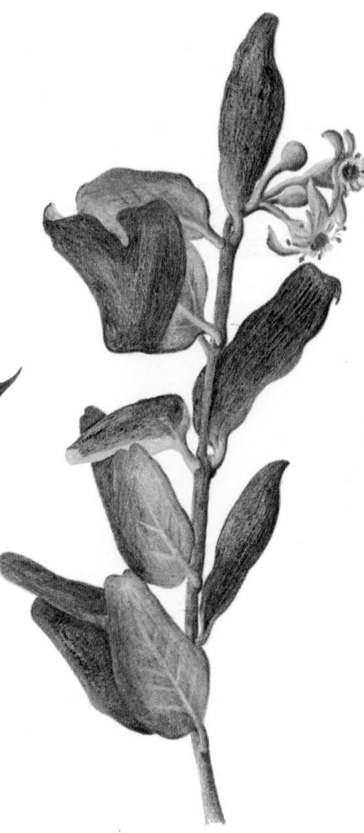

Make a tea from the leaves.

SERRALHA

Silybum marianum
Family: Compositae

The largest of the thistles. Found in the Amazon, as well as in Europe and North Africa.

Contains a substance which protects the liver. Also used as an antidote to poisoning, and to treat hemorrhoids. Can be used as a vaginal rinse.

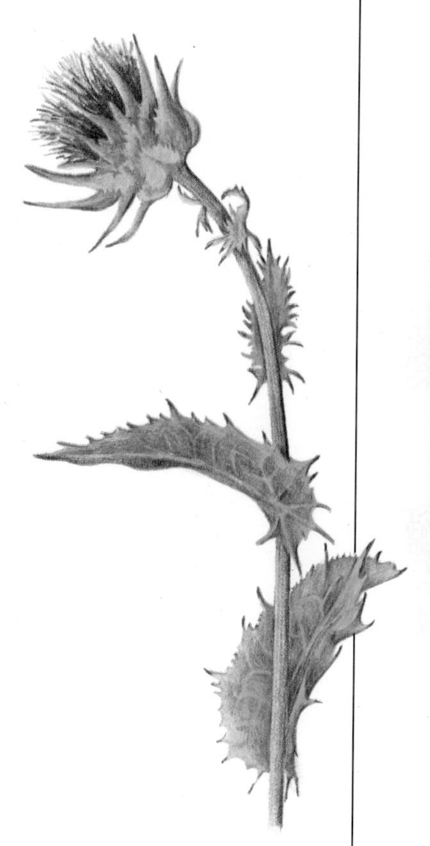

Make a tea from the fruit.

SARSAPARILLA

Smilax aspera
Family: Liliacae

Found on riverbanks throughout the Amazon.

Used to treat: Syphilis and all its complications, as well as various other sexually transmitted diseases, rheumatism, arthritis and arthrosis, various skin conditions, and hypercholesterolemia (excess cholesterol).

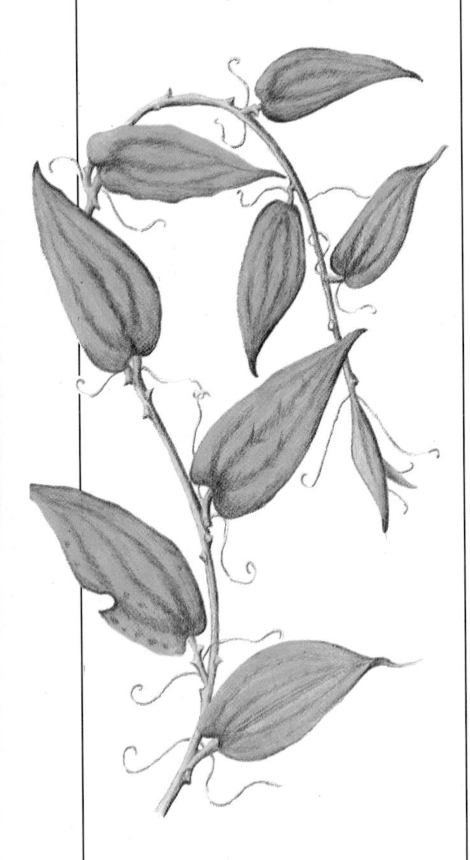

Use the leaves and roots. Make an infusion from the leaves, and or a decoction from the roots. The Indians make a soup from the roots and leaves.

DWARF NETTLE

Urtica urens
Family: Urticaceae

Found throughout the Amazon.

Used to treat: Anemia, tuberculosis, asthma, diabetes, hemophilia, gout, rheumatism, bleeding, and uremia. Often used for its anti-inflammatory properties.

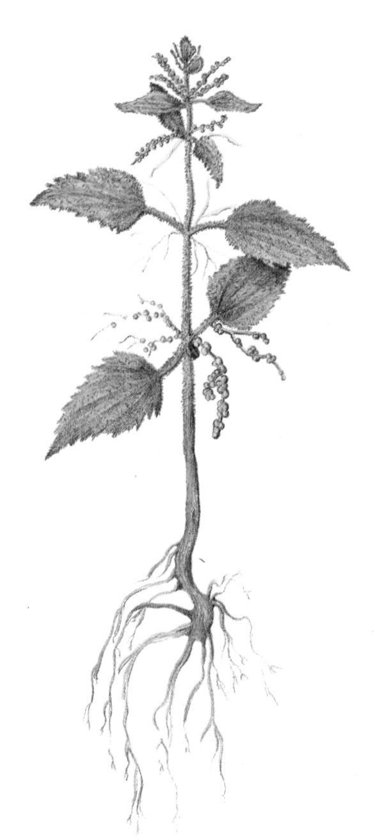

Make a tea from the leaves and flowers, or a decoction from the bark and roots. Boil for 10 minutes. The greens, which stimulate the digestive fluids and help prevent bladder deposits, can be used in a salad.

EUROPEAN VERVAIN, SPEEDWELL

Veronica officinalis
Family: Scrofulariaceae

Found throughout the Amazon.

Used to treat: Various conditions of the lungs and bronchial area, tuberculosis, gall-, kidney, and bladder stones, gout, and eczema. Also used as an antiseptic.

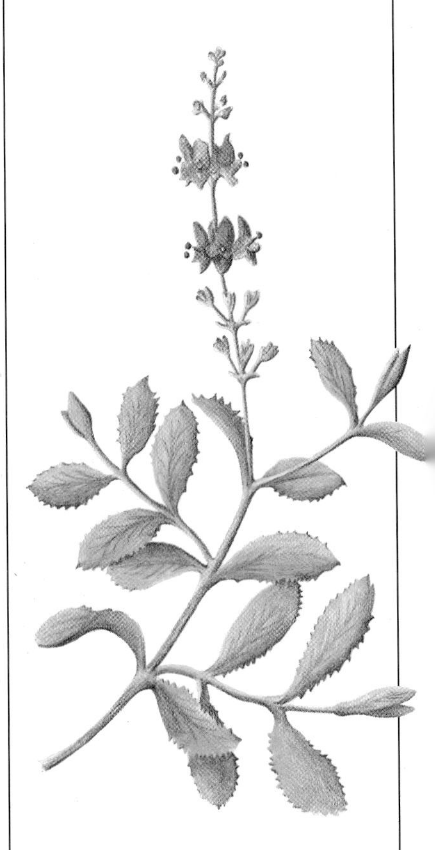

Use the entire plant. Use leaves and mature flowers to make a tea. Stems and branches can be used to make a decoction.

Medicinal Plants from the Far East

According to Dr. Li Qin,
University Clinic of Chengdu

Traditional Chinese medicine has been evolving for about five thousand years. Chinese traditional medicine directly influences the lives and dietary habits of the Chinese more so than most medical traditions. The Chinese have derived many health benefits from their practices, as statistics from the World Health Organization show year after year.

Thanks to the concepts of *yin* and *yang* (cold and warm), the Chinese have been aware for more than three thousand years that the therapeutic effects of plants are based on an interplay of components exercising both positive and negative influences. It took centuries to organize plants according to their yin and yang properties, but since then it has been relatively easy to apply this knowledge to everyday habits and nutrition. In cooking, for example, one must keep in mind that a meal with too much yang can have a detrimental effect on the yin organs (the kidneys, for example), and one can then change the nature of the meal in the method of preparation, say roasting vegetables instead of boiling them.

During my travels to the rainforests of China, I became convinced that there is no comparison to the variety of plants found in the Amazon, and that the Chinese plants did not possess the strength of the Amazon varieties because their environment is less harsh. But there are many important varieties that can be found only in Asia.

HUANG QI

Astragalus membranaceus
Family: Leguminosae

Found in the northern part of China.

Used primarily as a diuretic and as an immune booster. Has positive effects on the kidney and liver

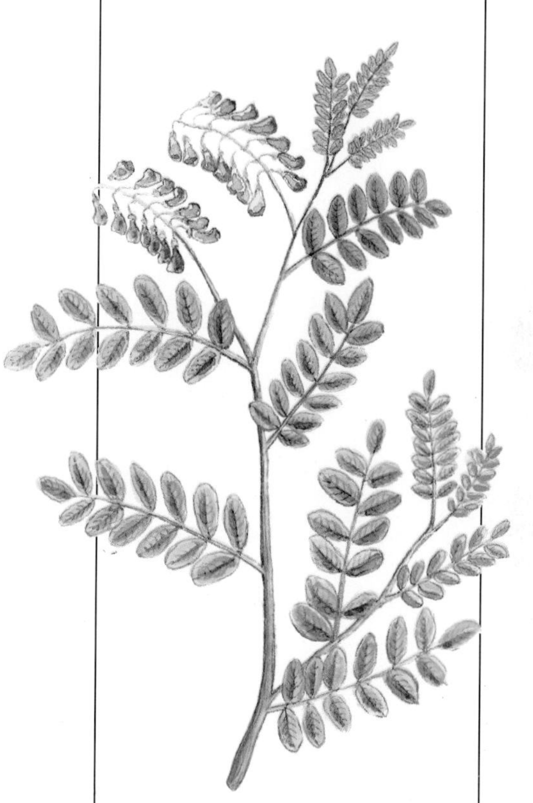

functions as well as hormonal balance, the heart, and circulation. Promotes kidney and skin circulation by dilating the capillaries. Lowers blood pressure and blood sugar.

Most effective when a decoction is prepared from the roots.

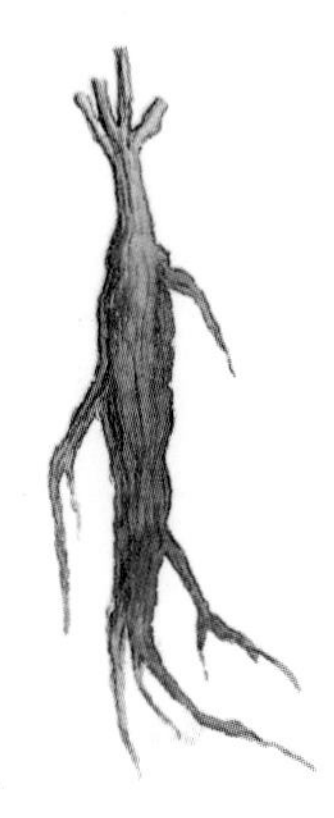

LONG YA CAO

Agrimonia pilosa
Family: Rosaceae

Found in China, Korea, and Japan.

Used to treat: Irregularities of the heart, liver, and lungs. Has coagulant and styptic properties. Used for all kinds of bleeding.

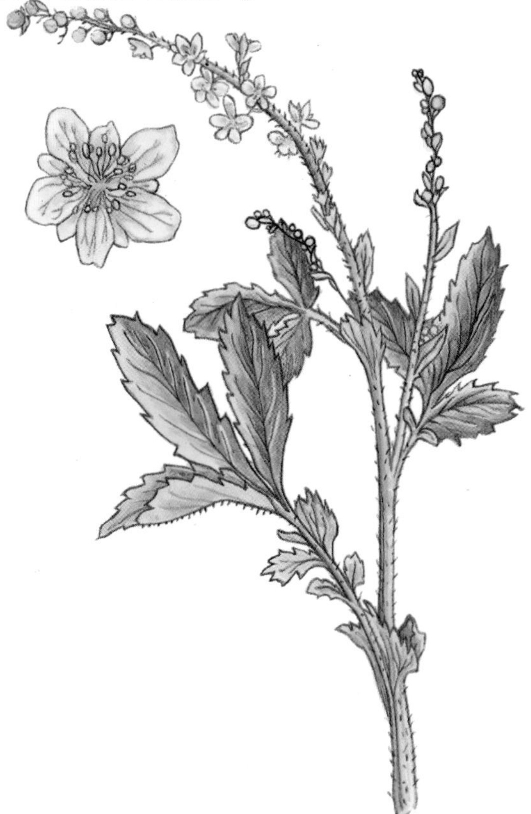

Extract enhances the production of thrombocytes.

Make an infusion from the leaves or a decoction from the roots.

For centuries, the Chinese have made a decoction from the branches to promote blood clotting and strengthen the osmotic resistance of blood vessels. Where these plants grow naturally, it's common to drink the decoction almost daily before meals.

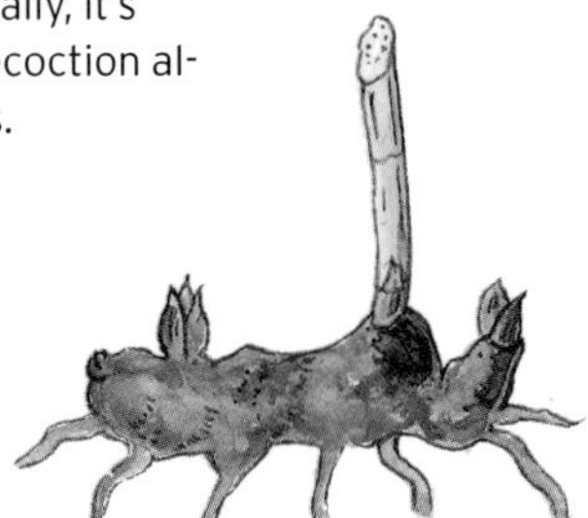

DU ZHONG

Eucommia ulmoides
Family: Eucommiaceae

Found only in China.

Used to treat: Liver and kidney insufficiency, lumbago, headache, impotence, and lumbago in pregnant women.

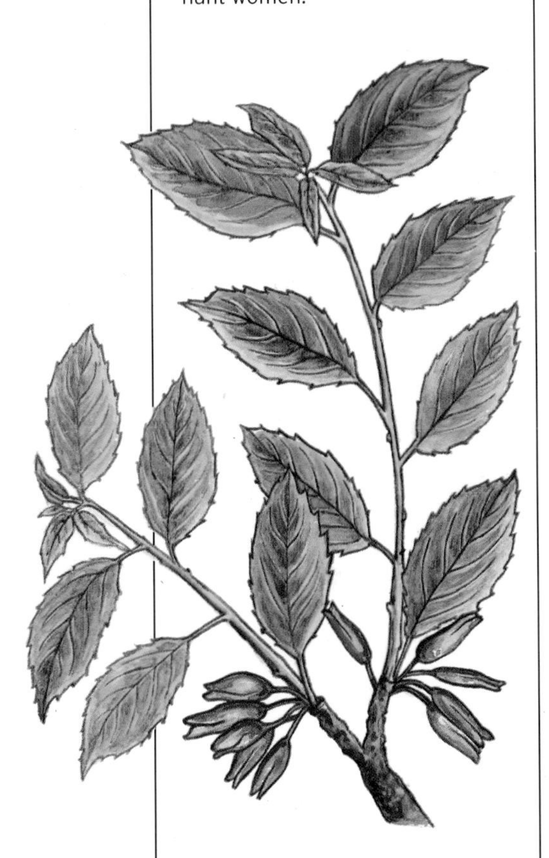

Make an extract from the bark.

WU JIA PI (SIBERIAN GINSENG)

Eleutherococcus gracilistylus
Family: Araliaceae

Found in China and Japan.

Used to treat: Rheumatism, arthritis, cramps, liver and kidney disfunction, and weakness in the back and legs. Beneficial for the liver and kidneys. Strengthens tendons and ligaments.

A tincture, which is made from the skin of the root and the branches, is said to increase sexual potency.

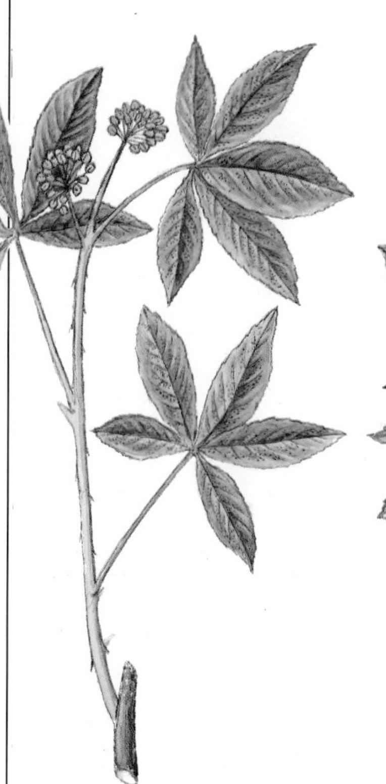

SAN QI (ASIAN GINSENG)

Panax notoginseng
Family: Araliaceae

Found in China and Japan.

Has positive effects on liver and stomach. Also used to reduce blood flow and release thrombocytes. It's styptic properties are best used by applying a tincture directly to an open wound. In most cases, the wound will heal without a scar.

The roots can be made into a decoction or tincture, or may be pulverized into a powder.

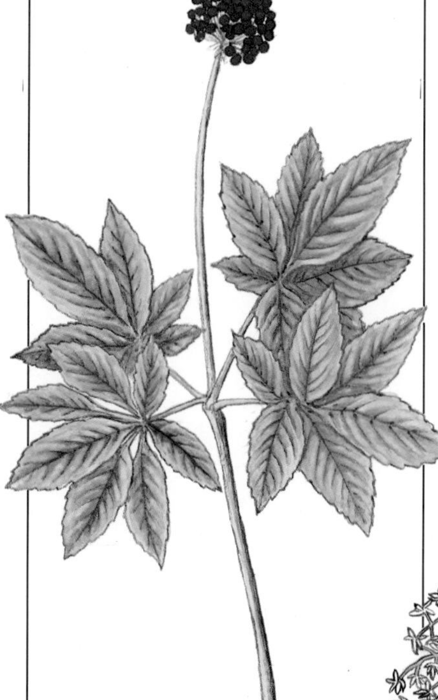

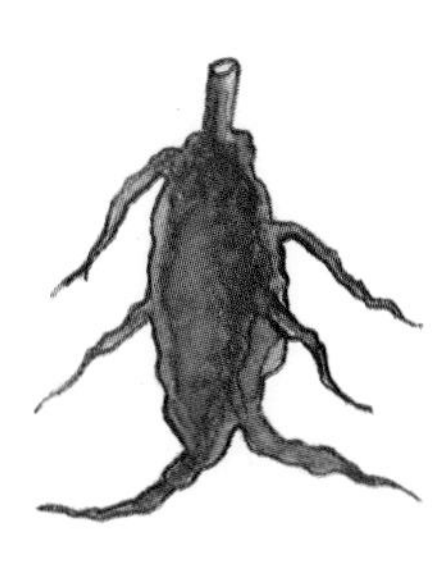

FO TI

Polygonum multiflorum
Family: Polygonaceae

Found in the rainforests of South China.

Used to treat: Problems with bone formation, swelling of the lymph nodes, and abscesses. Also useful for regulating metabolism, and as an antibiotic.

Recent research has shown that a decoction of roots and branches can also be effective in treatment of high blood pressure and arteriosclerosis.

The leaves can be used to make an infusion.

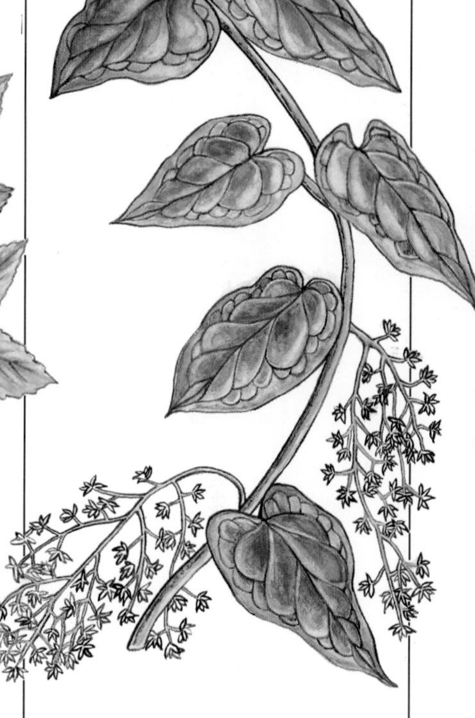

MA CHI XIAN

Portulaca oleracea
Family: Portulacaceae

Found only in China.

This plant is particularly beneficial for the colon and liver. It also relieves fever and helps remove toxins from the body. Used for anaerobic diarrhea, hemorrhoids, and abscesses.

The Chinese eat this plant as they would eat a vegetable. It works best when eaten fresh and can be taken in very high doses with no fear of side effects.

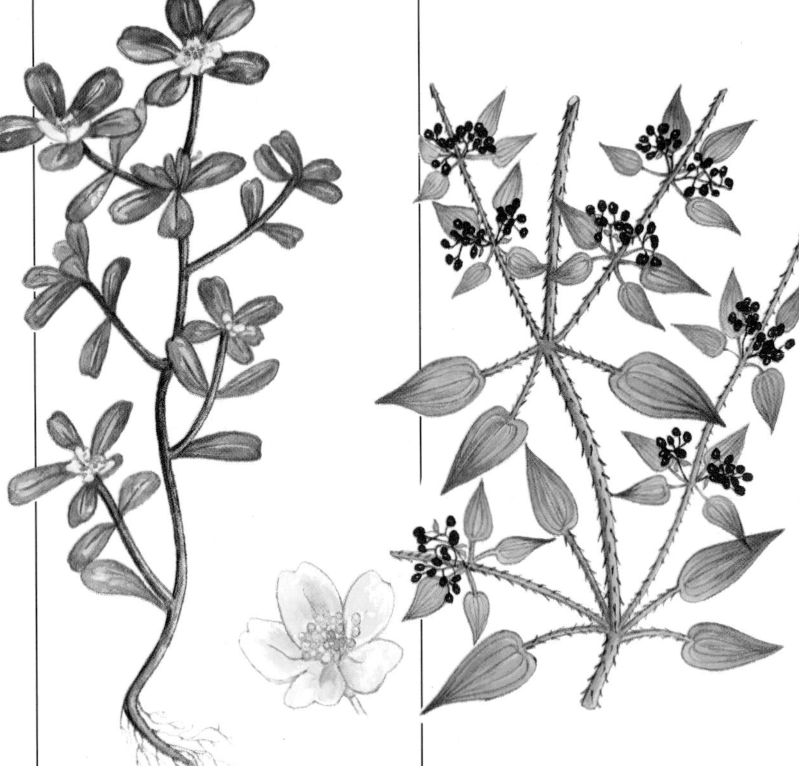

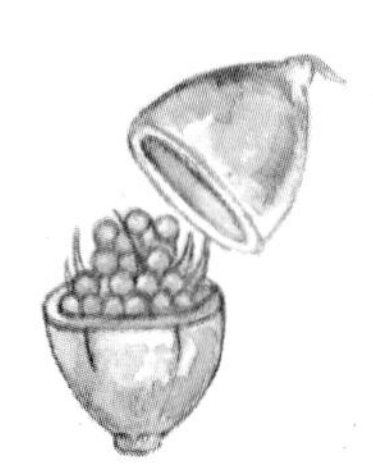

QIAN CAO GEN

Rubia cordifiola
Family: Rubiaceae

Found in China and Africa.

Releases the thrombocytes for arteriosclerosis and the triglycerides for high blood cholesterol.

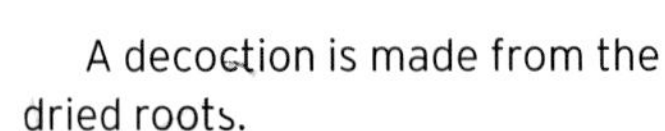

A decoction is made from the dried roots.

WU WEI ZI

Schisandra chinensis
Family: Magnoliaceae

Found in China and Japan.

Influences metabolism, regulates blood pressure, and provides a positive cardiovascular influence. Used to treat chronic coughs and asthma. The plant tends to dehydrate the organism, so take with plenty of fluids. But if the body does not have sufficient fluids, it serves to stimulate the mucous membranes and lubricates the organs.

An infusion is made from the dried berries.

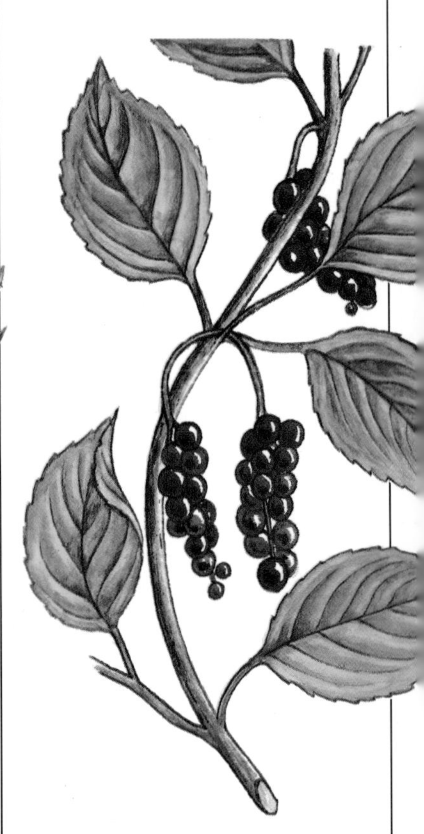

GOU TENG

Uncaria rhyncophylla
Family: Rubiaceae

Found in the south of China.

Works to relieve fever, calms the liver, and eases cramps. Take to treat headache, vision problems, and various cramps, especially for children. Helps ease discomfort in the sixth to eighth month of pregnancy.

A decoction made from the branches and needles opens up the capillaries and blood vessels, and also lowers blood pressure. Antimycotic, antibacterial, and antiviral effects are also mentioned in folk medicine.

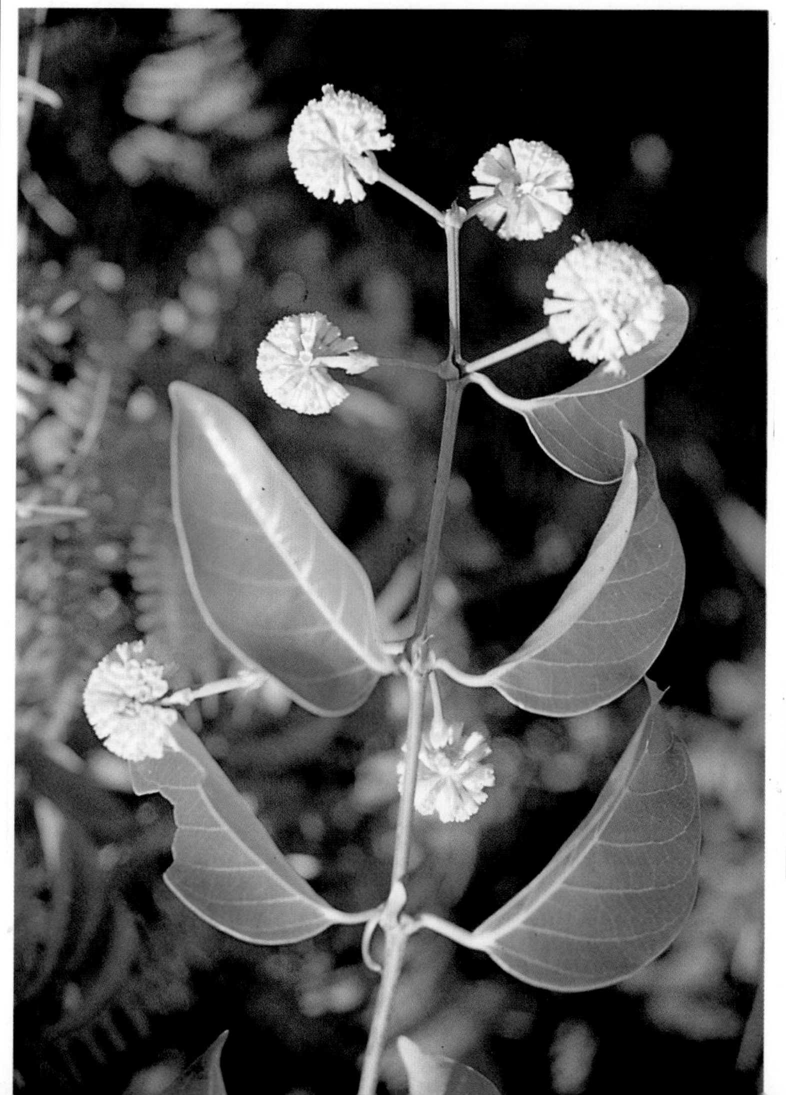

BAN ZHI LIAN

Scutellaria barbata
Family: Labiaceae

Found in China and Japan.

Used to treat: Abscesses, snake bite, bloated stomach, lung problems, and intestinal difficulties. Reduces fever and is used for its

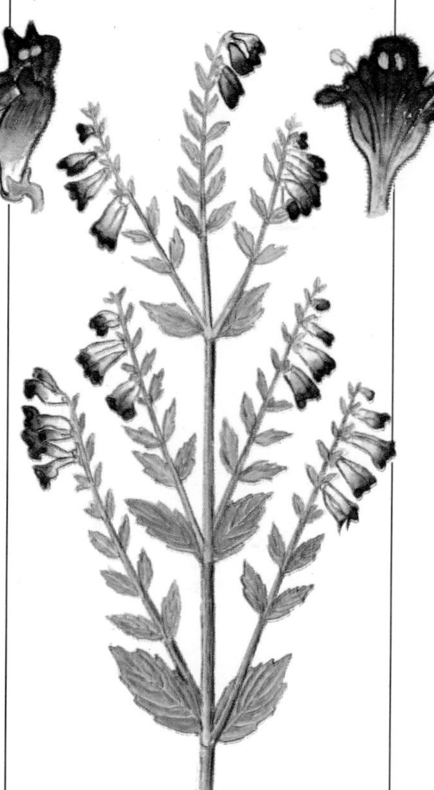

detoxifying, diuretic, styptic, and anti-inflammatory qualities.

The whole plant is used to make an infusion.

Nature in Your Own Backyard

One day, our own traditions of botanical medicine may provide replacements for the unbelievably hard-to-find components of CoD Rainforest Tea, but these unique and precious resources have yet to be replicated. If, however, a suitable substitute for these ingredients were to be found, it would ultimately benefit all those involved.

Production costs of working in and with the rainforest would decrease considerably, and harvesting and delivery would not be as much of a logistical nightmare.

BURDOCK

Arctium lappa
Family: Compositae

Grows to between 1 and 1½ meters high. Found in China, Japan, and North America, as well as Europe.

Benefits the lungs, stomach, kidneys, and liver. Strengthens kidney functions and helps remove toxins. A salve made from the burrs is used to prevent hair loss. The leaves contain tannin and traces of an essential oil, both of which have been proven effective against kidney stones and gallstones.

Use the roots, seeds, and leaves. Seeds and leaves are used to make an infusion. Roots can be used to make a decoction.

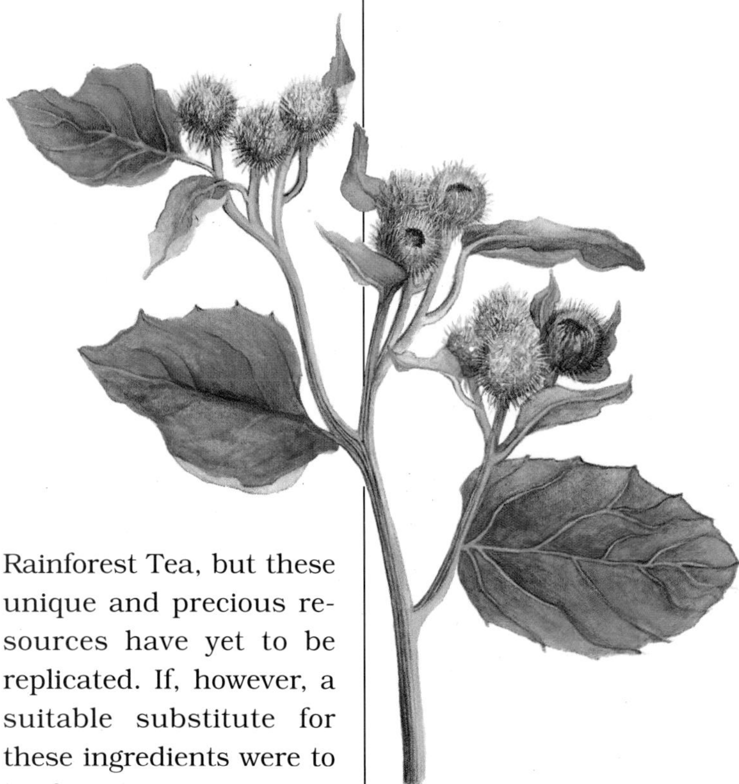

ST. JOHNSWORT

Hypericum perforatum
Family: Guttiferaceae

Found in South America and Europe. A shrub with a forked stalk and golden yellow flowers.

The tea, used to relieve stomach and intestinal discomfort, also helps relieve high blood pressure, digestive difficulties, internal and external bleeding, kidney and gall bladder complaints. Can be used externally to treat skin conditions and difficult-to-heal wounds. Used in a mouthwash, can be used to treat throat irritation and receding gums.

The tea is often used as an antidepressant.

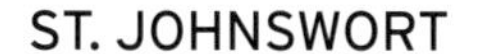

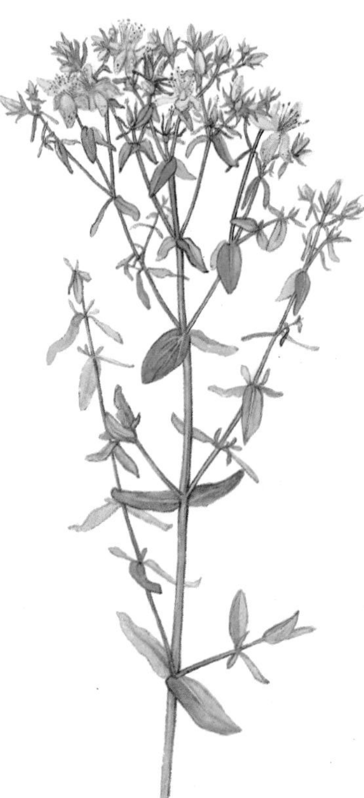

MINT

Mentha piperita
Family: Labiaceae

Found in Guyana, Surinam, China, and Europe.

Used to treat: Asthma, jaundice, liver deficiency, stomach ache, digestive difficulties, cramps, worms,

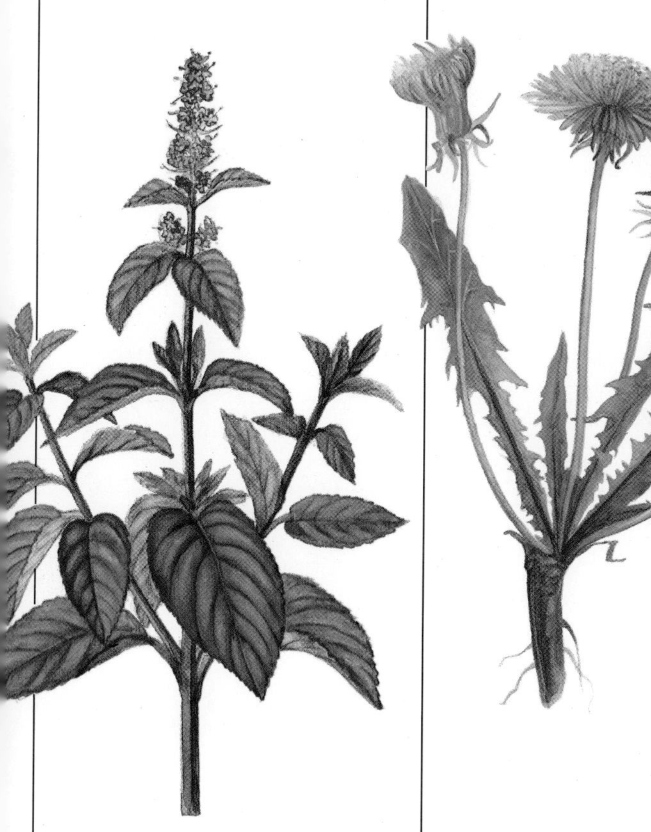

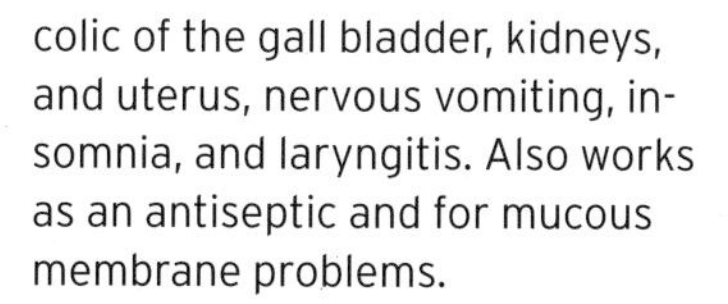

colic of the gall bladder, kidneys, and uterus, nervous vomiting, insomnia, and laryngitis. Also works as an antiseptic and for mucous membrane problems.

Make an infusion from the leaves and flowers.

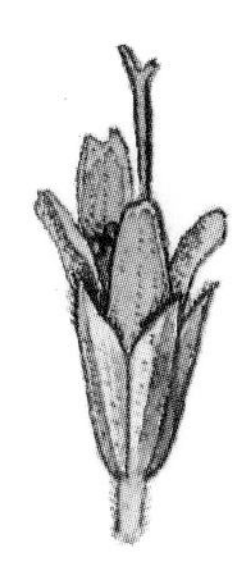

DANDELION

Taraxacum officinale
Family: Compositae

Found in the Amazon, China, and Europe.

Used to treat: Loss of appetite, hepatitis, liver deficiency, cholecystitis, diabetes, nephritis, and inflammation of the spleen. Especially helpful in reducing cholesterol and bile levels. Relieves gout and pain associated with rheumatism.

Also used as a diuretic or laxative.

The Indians eat this as a green.

EUROPEAN MISTLETOE

Viscum album
Family: Loranthaceae

Found in China and Central Europe.

Lowers blood pressure, relieves cramps and spasms, and has styptic properties. Also used to treat arthrosis and arteriosclerosis. Has

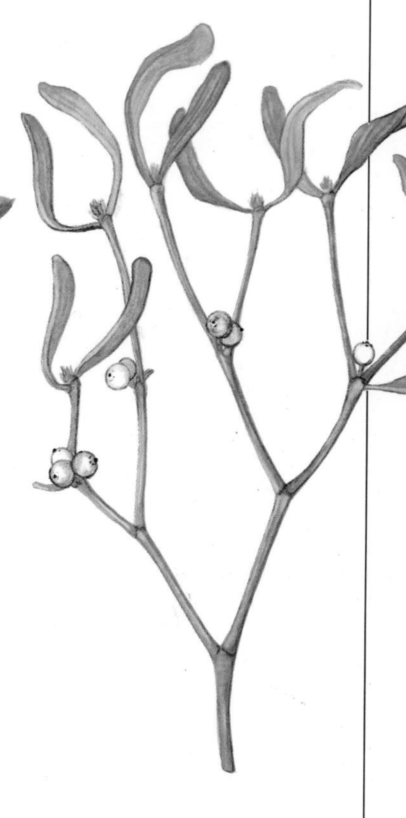

an immune-enhancing effect.

The white, pea-sized fruits are used, as well as the leaves and branches.

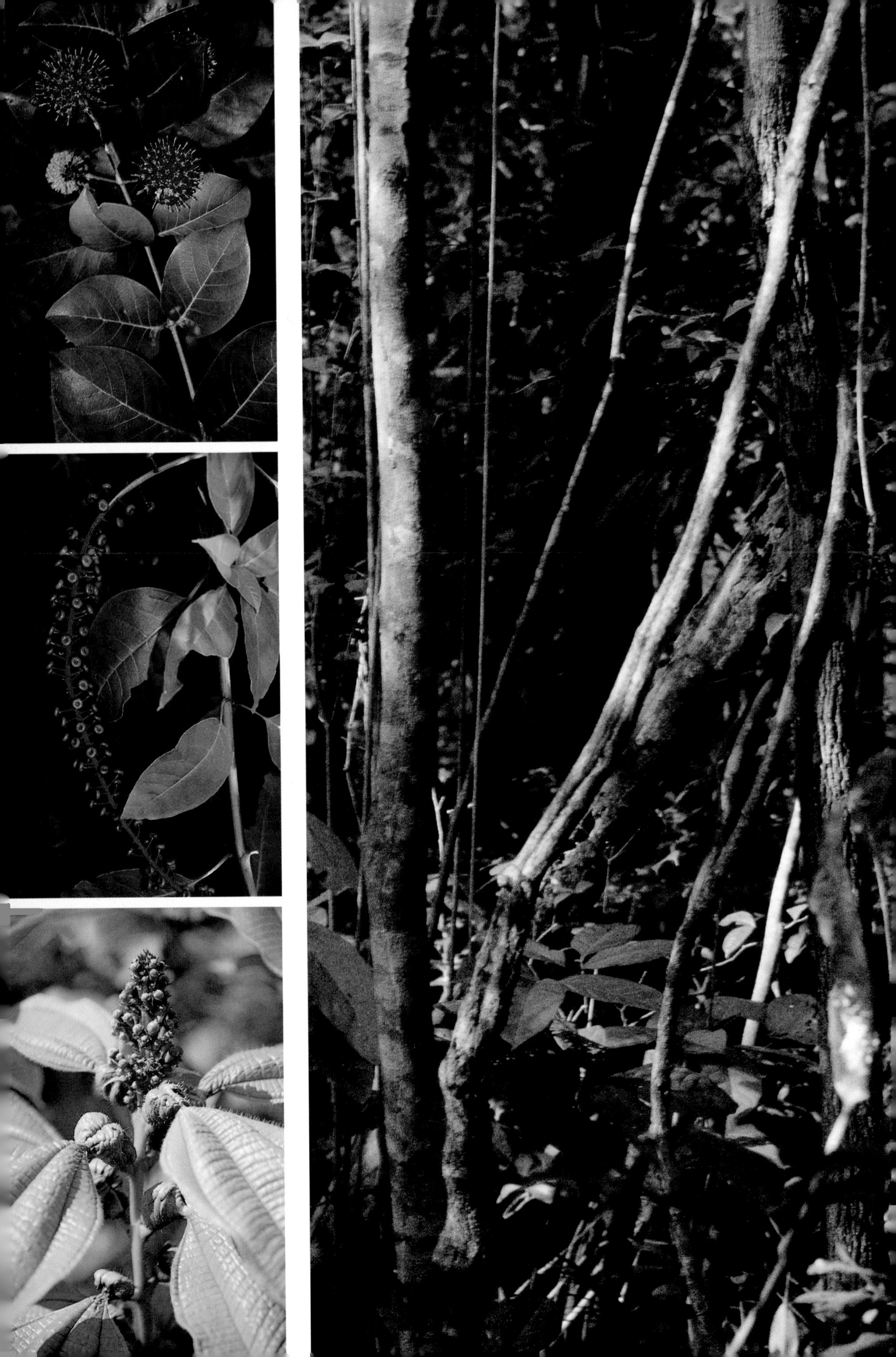

Plants: Stronger than Disease

Katunka continued his lecture. "I have learned from my father that all power and all life come from the forest. This life," he gestured toward the neatly arranged plants on the ground, "is stronger than disease."

Then Katunka showed me a few plants and explained the uses and effects of each of them. At first I recognized the symptoms he described in only a few cases. For example, if a child is having asthma symptoms (in general, most native children have bronchitis to some extent due to inhaling smoke from the open Maloka fire which burns throughout the night to drive away mosquitoes), I learned that Katunka would prescribe *alequin* for asthma and (just as his grandmother would) he would sit his patient in front of a pot of boiling water and have him or her inhale a decoction of eucalyptus.

But during the course of his lesson, it became difficult to distinguish between such conditions as high blood pressure and heart arrhythmia. That was harder.

Luckily, Katunka was a wonderful artist, and could depict all the human organs. He knew all about bronchial passages, and felt my prostate by pressing against my lower abdominal cavity. He pressed hard against my liver, which led me to understand that he was talking about hepatitis.

In the forest, he showed me which leaves and which pieces of bark were from which trees and bushes. He explained that the forest was poor, but very big. I didn't understand at first, but, thanks to many gestures, I finally understood. I looked around carefully. If you looked closely, you could see that there weren't as many varieties of plants as might be expected. The area was dominated by the trees and plants of the undergrowth. Katunka explained that sometimes he would send members of the tribe into the forest to look for specific varieties. Most of the varieties they needed could be found near the many rivers which crossed the area.

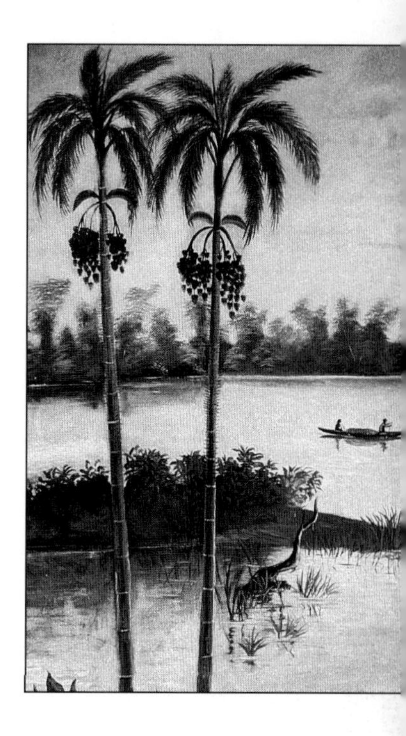

Feather drawing done by a native. While the Indians still find photos somewhat suspect, many of them are quite skilled at drawing and painting.

Opposite: The rainforest offers a startling variety of plants which have evolved into specific ecological niches.

The tribe had built a small hut to serve as a tribal "pharmacy." It was just tall enough that you could stand up inside, without bumping your head on the thatched ceiling, which was held aloft by twelve bamboo shafts.

Much later, I learned that the number twelve has special significance for the Indians. Even though the details differ from tribe to tribe, they all see themselves as an integral part of infinite Nature and the cosmos, with which they are one. All things, the visible and the invisible, are divided into six realms.

In the center is the Earth, with everything that grows and lives on it, with Heaven above and the Underworld below. Six directions determine the orientation of the living and the dead: North, South, East, West, Above, and Below. For example, the Earth realm has six paths, or exits, one in each direction. They are held up by twelve posts, which are the model for those that hold up the roof of the Maloka. In the view of most Indians, the Earth realm was created by the Great Shaman, a woman who has no name, or perhaps one whose name was never given to me. The power of the Great Shaman can be good or bad, spiritual or material.

Fruits, for example, grow from the menstrual blood of the Great Shaman (the Great Mother). If an intruder or some creature of the forest, such as a jaguar, eats a fruit, it takes on the evil power of the Great Shaman's menstrual blood.

The evil from this blood forces its way into the Maloka, upsetting the eternal natural balance of life. Warriors are called upon to protect this balance and, to avoid the penetration of the blood of the Great Mother, they must kill these jaguars and intruders. A tribal shaman's function is to drive away the evil spirits of intruders who have not yet been taken to the death realm. Again, I was reminded of how important it was for our expedition and for our life here with the Indians that we had been invited, and had not tried to force ourselves upon the Indians.

Men also enter into the creation story of the Indians. They impregnated the Great Mother Shaman so she could give birth to the Earth. The power of men is only good. Plants were created from the leftover sperm. These plants are only good, even though some are poisonous. One must learn to use this poison correctly.

But back to Katunka's pharmacy. Twelve bamboo poles held up the roof. Two opposing walls were made of thickly

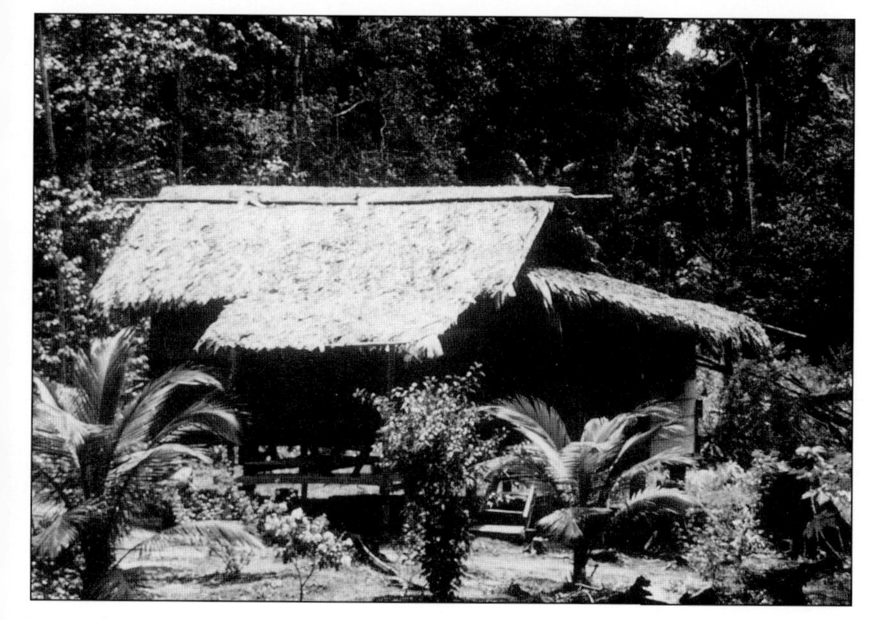

The jungle pharmacy, Katunka's pride and joy: filled with neatly ordered samples of tree bark, leaves, roots, and dried berries, and having a natural ventilation system to prevent mold and a unique, indescribable healing scent. As I clicked the shutter of my camera, Katunka asked me for the first time not to take any photographs. Evidently he believed that the camera might work some kind of bad magic on the healing powers of the plants.

braided mats. The other two walls were made from earthen bricks which were staggered to form a sort of checkerboard pattern with numerous openings that allowed for constant air circulation. Katunka explained to me, almost as an aside, that any mold on the plants would reduce their potency.

I had no idea at the time how important this method of storing the plants would be for me in the future in bringing plants from here to Europe. Instead, I just enjoyed (a bit too lustfully) the aromas of this herb dispensary like the scent of a summer morning. It was also wonderful that there were no mosquitoes in the room. Not a single insect was lurking, waiting to drill through the layers of my skin and taste my blood. Perhaps the most pleasurable thing about this room was that I could breathe freely. There was no trace of the constant mosquito-repelling smoke of the Maloka.

Although hunting is specifically and exclusively the domain of the men, and agriculture is "women's work," Katunka took me to his tribe's garden. It was the sorriest looking little garden I'd ever seen. Just beyond it there was some undergrowth a good ten meters high, with trees up to forty-five meters in height towering above. There were a few tree stumps in the field, and there was some ash on the ground to lend some paltry nourishment to the soil and a few plants.

They grew manioc, green beans which they call "phisolo" (which actually originated here in South America), bananas, some herbs, cotton, and tobacco. I saw a few gourds here and there. The plants looked wretched, but some of the gourds themselves must have weighed fifty pounds.

Five thousand years ago, our European ancestors practiced the same kind of slash-and-burn agriculture. But there was a difference: in Europe, even after a large field had been burned, it would remain productive. That is not the case in the Amazon.

Researchers have proven that the fertility of the Amazon stems from the climate, not from the soil. Here, the essential nutrients necessary for the plants to thrive are found in the plants themselves, and not in the soil. The soil serves mostly to anchor the plants down.

It follows that the large-scale burning of forests and fields which threaten the Amazon and the world climate is completely insane. We are burning down the only thing of value: the plants and trees. The soil is probably able to absorb some of the nutrients, but these will more than likely be depleted after the first harvest. It's as if a bank robber has burned all the money he's stolen in order to make more money out of the ashes.

On a later trip to the Amazon, I was able to see the price to be paid by those who ignore the rules of the jungle. In the middle of a huge field in Brigantina I saw ten thousand hectares of forest that had been burned down. Settlers had come from the slums of the city to build small farm houses.

The soil held out for five years. Now the land is barren. The houses are empty, and several hundred of them were not even finished when the builders discovered that the soil would not provide for them.

An even more senseless crime against the rainforest (due to its magnitude) was the building of a road which would have circled the area. Today the road is impassable most of the year, except for commercial trucks and tractors, which cannot negotiate the road in any season.

I have heard that there once was a massive flood while the road was still under construction. In one place, where there were a dozen tractors and graders, the road was completely washed out. The tractors are still rusting there today, and the workers either fled into the forest or drowned.

The Indians do things very differently. Everything they do is on a scale appropriate to their needs. They don't need to be convinced that "Small is beautiful." This slogan, or its intent, is part of their tradition and the way they live their lives, and they remain true to it.

I could see that Katunka was proud of the garden. He said, "There is power in plants. When we eat these plants, they give us this power, just as Epena gives us the spirit."

Epena is a drug used by the Yanomamo which, when taken in small amounts, enhances the senses. To Katunka, this was the power of the spirit.

"And what about animals?" I asked.

"They make us full," he said, as if hunger was an illness, and meat was simply a remedy.

Already after my first lesson with Katunka, I could follow his words more easily, while before, in the hospital in Sao Paulo, I could only understand his "thank you" speech (which he had evidently practiced). That night, I drove myself crazy wondering how Katunka and the Yanomamo could distinguish six from seven and twelve from thirteen. I had read (and later confirmed that it was true) that the Yanomamo, and other Amazon tribes, could only count to three, and anything more was simply "a lot."

Nevertheless their worldview consisted of six levels, with exits held aloft by twelve posts. Katunka explained this to me in Portuguese. Would an average member of the tribe be able to distinguish between three and four, or between nineteen and twenty?

"No," said Alton.

Young Suma, aka Thomas, came slinking by. It seemed he wanted some more peppermint candy.

"Close your eyes," I said, and showed him what I meant.

Suma closed his eyes and squealed with delight. He knew too well the sound of the little container in which I stored sugary things which had become sticky and gooey. I flipped over an aluminum pot and scattered ten pieces of candy on the bottom.

"How many do you see, Suma?" I asked.

He was very excited. "A lot."

"Now put your hands in front of your eyes, and don't peek," I said, as I silently took one away. "How many do you see now?"

Suma took his hands away, opened his eyes, and looked somewhat disappointed. Without skipping a beat, he said, "There's one missing."

We repeated the game, this time with small, round slices of the pumpernickel bread we had brought with us. They weren't so sweet looking, and were far less appealing to Suma than the peppermint candies, so he could be a more objective subject. Regardless of whether I put down thirty and took away two, or put down ten and added three, Suma knew at a glance, without counting, whether I had added to the slices or taken some away. I was convinced: Suma was a mathematical genius. He was best with amounts, but had no words for numbers. I was convinced that I could have taught him to add, subtract, multiply, and divide within a few weeks, and thought I might do so on a subsequent visit.

Unfortunately, it was not to be. Suma grew up to be a real troublemaker and hooligan, and he let me know, in no uncertain terms, that he held no affection for whites, including me. To Suma, the only good thing about us was the kazoo that Freddy gave him as a good-bye present after our first trip.

Learning and Planning

With every lesson, it became clearer to me that there is something ever present and unique about botanical medicine. Katunka's knowledge had many similarities with customs that wise and knowledgeable Chinese have shared with me, which are in turn similar to the knowledge of the practical Styrian farmer, or to the wisdom of the ancient herbal remedies of Provence.

I assumed that even the ancient Indo-Germanic and Celtic peoples had their own shamans. For the moment, though, I did not have the opportunity to investigate these questions further. During my first visit, I decided I would have Katunka's plants thoroughly analyzed and tested.

This project would soon become my life. During the next several years, I had to struggle to keep my animal clinic in Vienna from going under, for the most part without actually being there.

The shaman had described to me the ability of the plants to heal an ailment which I suspected was what we in Europe call cancer. It would be some time before I could test this and we could establish a reliable system of transport and supply. When I had become more familiar with the plants, and the zones in which they are to be found, it became clear to me that I would have to visit other tribes who made their homes along the rivers of the Amazon. I would meet many people during this early phase. Most were of great help to me, while others, whom

I had known for years, tried to trip me up.

I am obligated to thank everyone who was involved, those who helped as well as those who tried to hinder the project. Looking back, I am convinced that even the obstacles contributed to the success of the project. For example, at the airport in Belem, a customs inspector gave me a good tongue-lashing because I had packed a couple of plants in my bags. I conceded that this was true. I was smuggling nature treasures, a crime, plain and simple.

A government official witnessed my scolding, and on the plane to Frankfurt I explained to him why I wanted to take the plants with me. He advised me to have the Indians send them to me in the future. They have the right to send a package to any part of the world without any kind of export clearance. It wasn't as simple as it sounded, but it did open the way for me to successfully have plants sent to Europe without jumping through bureaucratic hoops each step of the way.

On the day of my departure from the Maloka, Katunka put his hands on my shoulders and said, "I am old. Will I see you again?"

Since then I've seen him once a year, which is as often as I visit my mother in Canada.

"And what about the garimpeiros?" I asked him worriedly.

"They will not find us. They are cowards. If you chase them and kill one of them, the others run away like chickens."

I had learned, as the first tangible results of this trip, the

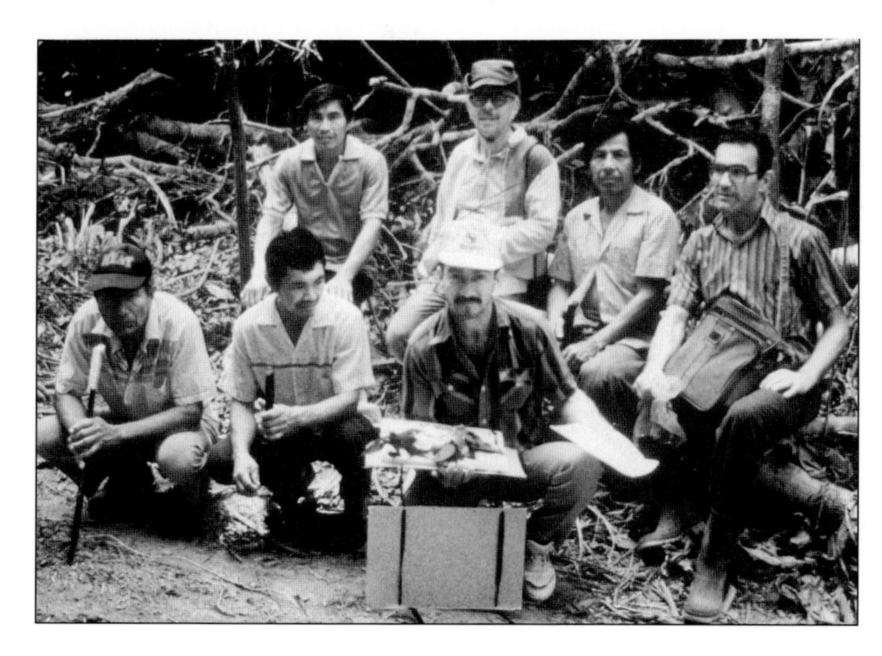

Collectors at rest: German tropical medicine specialist, Dr. Oliver Gyulavari *(front right)* with assistants.

basics of the shamans' botanical medicine. I sketched out a table and wrote down some of the details of my newfound knowledge on my flight to Europe. Since then, the list of plants has grown much longer, but at least a fifth of what I've learned I owe to my first lessons with Katunka.

First Clinical Proof

Arriving in Vienna, I examined the plants which Katunka had given me. It was clear that I would have to put them through an endless series of biochemical and toxicological tests before I could do anything else. As a basis for these tests, I wanted to concentrate on the mixture that Katunka had given me to treat the so-called jungle fever. We had to know beyond a shadow of a doubt that the mixture was in no way poisonous. Certainly I trusted the knowledge and experience of the millenia-old tradition of the shamans, but my convictions alone would not be sufficient.

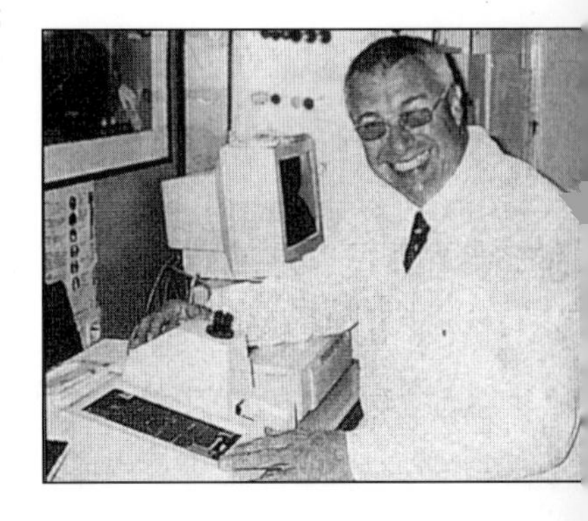

Clinical tests: I was extremely fortunate that specialists volunteered their time and skills. Without their selfless assistance, I would have been forced to give up the project for lack of funding.

Dr. Harald Greger, a world-renowned ethnobotanist and Director of the Institute of Comparative Botanical Studies in Vienna, was extremely helpful in guiding this part of the work. He arrived at essentially the same results as those which, years later, the Austria Foodstuffs Research Institute discovered under the direction of Dr. Werner Pfanhauser.

Before I could give the plants over for testing, I needed to find a name for the mixture. I had brought them to Europe in a jute bag, which customs had stamped "CoD." I had no time to waste thinking up creative names, and had already used the term "CoD" with my colleagues as a working name, so I decided to go with "CoD Tea."

On April 9, 1996, I received the results. Here is the final report:

"After thoroughly researching all the information submitted to us, and the relevant literature, we have come to the following conclusions on your CoD Tea:

"CoD Tea is best when prepared in boiling water, and ingested in a manner similar to that of an herbal tea. We were able to determine at the time of preparation that the mixture in question is of little nutritional value, and is not necessarily to be consumed for taste or enjoyment. Since this preparation, according to our observation and analysis, is of little or no pharmaceutical value, it should therefore be regulated as an edible consumer product according to the Austrian Foodstuffs Law of 1975. This law stipulates that importation or marketing (including, but not limited to, announcements and advertising) of this product cannot be made in connection to any claims as to its therapeutic value, even when such claims create the impression that consumption of the preparation will create beneficial results of a physiological nature.

"Before marketing edible consumer products, the marketer must first register with the Austrian Ministry of Health and Consumer Protection.

"The following amendment must be made to the above results, with respect to the drug scopolamine: scopolamine is related to and shares some similarities with a substance known as coumarin. In regard to its properties as a plant-growth inhibitor, there is some evidence in the literature for the potential of toxic effects. We see no evidence, however, in regard to the product in question, of potential negative side effects. Nonetheless, we recommend that CoD Tea be marketed only with the stipulation that the amount of scopolamine (and coumarin) content should in no way exceed 2 milligrams per liter of finished product."

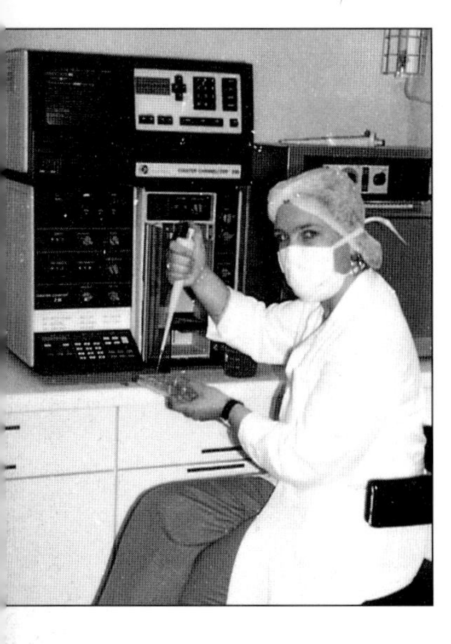

Components of the tea were thoroughly analyzed according to the latest scientific methods in order to detect any possible harmful ingredients. Today the tea is tested regularly to guarantee purity and consistent quality.

Coumarin is a naturally occurring and very common glycoside. In our area it's found in woodruff and other plants. According to the Brockhaus Encyclopedia, it has a "very pleasant aroma and taste." It's manufactured synthetically in the fragrance industry and used in great quantities as an indispensable fragrance for hay and lavender scents, and for tobacco. It can cause damage to the kidneys in very high concentrations, but the concentrations found in CoD Tea tested far below this level. If coumarin is, in fact, responsible for the effects of the tea, we have yet to determine to what extent. We know which plants contain it. But because we were following a recipe that has been used for millennia, we didn't want to change it and reduce its effectiveness. So we decided not to take anything out of the recipe and at the same time remain within the prescribed limits of coumarin content.

As I said, this report was from 1996. The events I'm describing took place in 1983. In between lay thirteen years of phyto- and biochemical research, with friends and colleagues selflessly volunteering their services simply because they had a genuine interest in the project. In addition to Dr. Greger, I would also like to thank Magister Briggitte Brem, a world-class biochemist, Dr. Otmar Hofer, Head of Analytical Chemistry at the University of Vienna, and Dr. Peter Galfi, biochemist at the University of Budapest. Dr. Galfi was the first to undertake longterm studies and observe and document the effects of the tea on healthy and pathogenic cells. In the spring of 1987 lab test results were convincing enough to give me confidence to try the tea out on animals with terminal diseases.

There were plenty of four-legged creatures in my clinic with cancer or AIDS.

These animals had terminal illnesses, a very short life expectancy, and a thoroughly painful existence. I needed only the permission of the owners before I could begin to help these poor creatures find a little comfort in their lives.

As chance would have it, my three-year-old cat, Doktor Doc, had just developed a malignant tumor. I operated on him, and gave him the tea after the operation, which I administered with a pipette. In four weeks, my beloved Doc was up and around. Contrary to the normal course of tumor treatment, no metastases formed after surgery.

I had every reason to expect these results, but I still felt as if I had witnessed a miracle. Today I have some more plausible explanations and much more knowledge on the positive effects of the rainforest plants. One essential part of this knowledge I owe to Derek Proctor, a cancer patient.

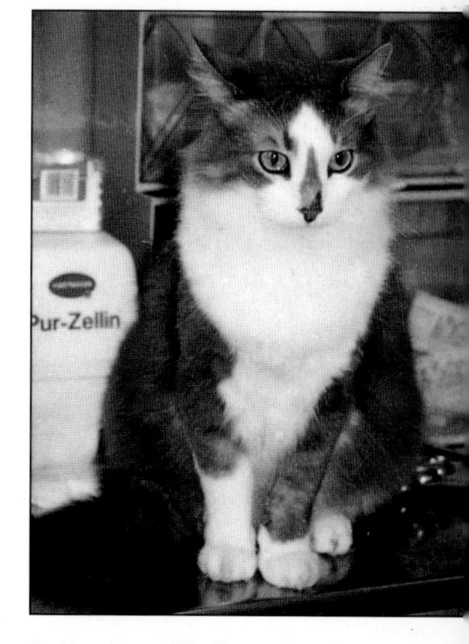

Doktor Doc, still alive and well, has lived to a ripe old age.

Derek Proctor lives in Bangkok, where he became ill. Doctors diagnosed him as having liver cancer. After having a tumor removed in surgery, Derek sold all his belongings and returned to his Irish homeland. His son had somehow heard of my tea and told his father about it. At the end of 1995, I received a letter in which Derek described his situation as "hopeless," and he asked me if I would provide him with a month's supply of tea. I was glad to do so. When the month was up, he asked me for another month's supply, because he thought he felt an improvement in his condition. Based on my experience with Derek, I developed an extensive correspondence with Dr. Reimar Bruening of Myco Pharmaceuticals in Cambridge, Massachusetts.

Among other things, Dr. Bruening quoted a letter from Proctor's son, dated May 1, 1996:

"My father's condition has improved. He has gained eight pounds, and is also much stronger. Now he can walk around without help, which we could only dream of as recently as a few months ago. Naturally, I don't want to entertain the hope that he's cured or that his metastases are in total remission, but every day that he lives is a miracle, and he's already survived much longer than the four months his doctor gave him. Thankfully, he's not in any pain. While it's impossible to know the cause of his improvement, I firmly believe that taking CoD Tea has played a significant role."

Also, by way of the U.S.A., I discovered the clinical work of Dr. Judah Folkman, a researcher at Harvard Medical School and Dr. Bruening's neighbor.

About twenty years ago, Dr. Folkman discovered that tumors have an unusually high concentration of blood vessels. Today, we know that this is because rapidly reproducing tumor cells need great amounts of oxygen.

Dr. Folkman determined that once a tumor has reached a critical mass, it begins producing a protein which halts the production of blood vessels. He isolated this protein, which is called angiostatin. What is fascinating is that angiostatin suppresses the production of metastases that are already present in the body. The stiff competition from the tumor and the angiostatin which it produces prevent metastases from developing.

This explanation was in line with previous studies. It often happens that six months, or in some cases longer, after the removal of a tumor metastases will develop in various parts of the body. Actually, these groups of metastases existed already. But once the tumor, and the source of metastases-suppressing angiostatin, is removed, they can develop without hindrance.

This theory was accepted by most cancer research centers in the U.S. Many of Dr. Folkman's colleagues are certain that one day he'll receive a Nobel Prize for his work.

On Dr. Bruening's recommendation, I studied Dr. Folkman's publications. I had learned of a fascinating six-month study he was undertaking, in which researchers implanted a tumor (carcinoma) in a group of rats. The rats were then divided into three groups. Two of the groups were treated with angiostatin while the third group received no treatment. None of the untreated rats survived, but the tumors in the other two groups disappeared within five to six weeks. The first group (of the two groups treated with angiostatin) was then treated with Endoxan, a substance used in chemotherapy, and the second group was untreated. The untreated group developed tumors again within two weeks. As this book goes to press, rats from the group treated with Endoxan are still alive and thriving. Dr. Folkman came to the following conclusions:

The protein angiostatin prevents the development of new blood vessels, allowing the body's natural immune system (which unfortunately can only kill tumor cells very slowly) to reduce the tumor to a microscopic size, at which time the oxygen supply to the tumor is too small to allow it to regenerate. This appears to be the appropriate stage to initiate cytotoxic chemotherapy in order to eradicate the remnants of the tumor cells. This is exactly what occurred in the case of the rats treated with Endoxan. Without the introduction of angiostatin to support the chemotherapy treatment, however, it is likely that any remaining tumor cells could rebound sufficiently to produce another life-threatening tumor.

Dr. Bruening had taken it upon himself to share with Dr. Folkman some similar results which had been achieved with CoD Tea. Dr. Bruening said, "He wasn't the least bit surprised. As a matter of fact, he thought it was probable that in addition to the immune boosters in the tea, there may be some component which has effects similar to those of angiostatin."

Happily, Dr. Folkman explained that he would research the effects of my tea. At present, we know what the effects are,

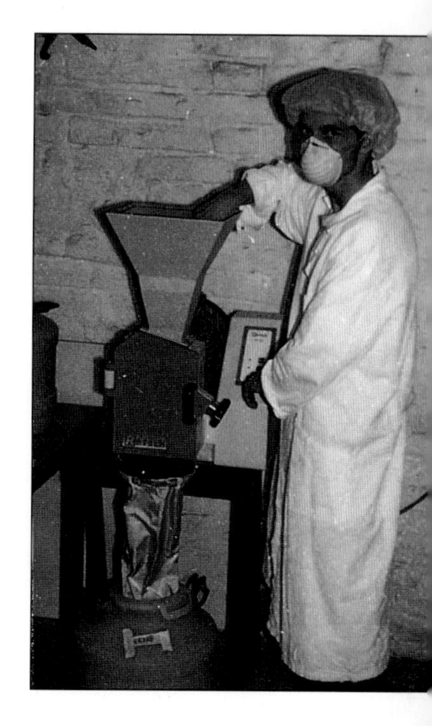

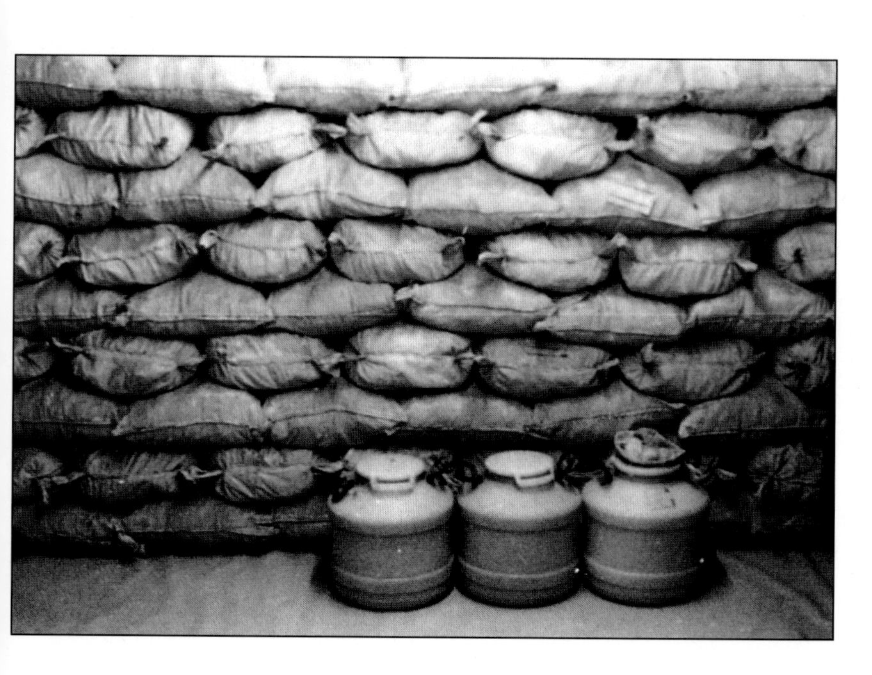

Constant concerns: safe, efficient transportation and storage. The tree bark used in the CoD Tea is so hard that special steel grinders had to be made in order to grind it economically. The shamans of the Amazon, who are normally not pressed for time, use the time-tested method of pounding the bark with hard stones.

but we don't fully understand the mechanisms which bring these effects into play.

The Greeks are convinced that botanical substances can have positive effects on both normal cells and "bad" cells (such as tumor cells). I have heard the story of an American who was afflicted with bladder cancer. In the intensive care unit, his American doctor had had a special oil prepared from some type of sage, which he injected directly into the patient's bladder. In a few weeks, the patient's tumor was in remission to such an extent that it couldn't be detected by X ray or CAT scan. Two years later, the patient was up and around and totally fit.

I haven't heard how he's doing today, and I cannot vouch that the story is totally true. I do, however, consider it worth mentioning that, while Greeks are convinced of the tumor-healing properties of sage oil, no one has yet made the effort to test this traditional cure.

In my correspondence with specialists throughout the world, I have also learned of a compound in Japan which has effects very similar to those of angiostatin, but which is unfortunately toxic.

This substance was derived from Fumagillin, a byproduct of a fungus. A biochemist asked me if it's possible that there is a microscopic fungus in CoD Tea which produces some kind of product like angiostatin, but without having any negative side effects.

Remarkable Results

Our work was cut out for us, but at least we had accomplished the most important goal: we had shown that CoD Tea, if used in conjunction with a sensible lifestyle and a prescribed diet, can lead to a notable improvement in overall well-being and quality of life for many patients with terminal cancer, without any harmful side effects.

I'd like to give details of this in the amazing results of three seemingly hopeless cases. Although these results are not typical for all patients, they nevertheless show the immense power that is concealed in these rainforest plants.

From examining patient's cases, I have determined the following:

- 46 percent responded that their condition is "no better, no worse."

- 38 percent reported a significant improvement in their condition, of which:
    - 31 percent responded that their condition is "better."
    - 60 percent responded that their condition is "much better."
    - 9 percent responded that their condition is "excellent."

I defined "excellent" as "remission of one or more tumors to such an extent that they can no longer be detected."

"Much better" was defined as "able to work, free of symptoms, and tumors have decreased in size as confirmed by X ray or ultrasound."

"Better" was defined as "mostly free of pain, better general condition, and able to gain weight."

This data is based on the interpretation of X rays, CAT scans, ultrasound tests, tumor markers, immune status, general examination findings from hospitals, clinics, and laboratories, and the subjective reports from patients and their physicians.

Based on the experiences and results, which we gained from more than two thousand terminal cancer patients, it is obvious in which cases the CoD method, as a complementary therapy, can support the protective and self-healing forces of the body: lung cancer, non-Hodgkin's lymphoma, breast cancer, bladder cancer, cancer of the large intestine, osteosarcoma, leukemia, metastasis of the lung, liver, brain, and bone, and chronic fatigue syndrome.

Before I begin describing the case studies, I'd like my readers to be aware of two things:

1. Many readers will not be familiar with some of the terminology in the following descriptions. For this reason, I've included a glossary at the back of the book.

2. All the case studies cited here are based on results obtained from work done with patients at various clinics. The patients described had already started a course of treatment before they began taking CoD Tea. These results have been forwarded to us voluntarily by either patients or their doctors, and they have been invaluable in our research. Patients are identified by first name and last initial only. Almost all two thousand patients have been willing to share their experiences with others, and such information can be obtained by

contacting us in Vienna at the address in the back of the book. The mother of a young patient with cancer of the lymph nodes began her correspondence like this:

"You can't imagine what I've been through the last few months. My son is doing so well that he's gone back to kindergarten, and is free of symptoms. I've thought about how I might possibly thank God for what has happened, and I realized that the least I can do is share our experiences involving your rainforest tea with other mothers and fathers who find themselves in similar situations. I remember distinctly how much I longed for such an exchange of information when my son started the treatment, but at that time there was no one available to share their experiences. After all I've been through, I have enough experience not to awaken any blind hopes, which can only lead to pain and sorrow if things don't work out for the best."

Case Studies

Ruth, age 4

Ruth is a four-year-old leukemia patient. In April 1995 she was admitted to a hospital in Vienna. She was given a bone marrow test and a battery of blood tests. Her weakened immune system led to an infection on the inside of her mouth, which first manifested itself as a hard lump. On May 8, preparations were made for a bone marrow transplant. On May 15, doctors learned that her siblings could not be considered as donors.

On May 18, she was treated with cortisone for a high fever. Ruth's blood count: leukocytes 7,000 (normal levels range from 7,000 to 10,000), and thrombocytes 103,000 (normal value: 300,000).

After the cortisone treatment, Ruth's condition improved at first. It was determined that the cause of her mouth infection was the HI-6 virus (a form of herpes). Blood levels worsened to leukocytes 4,700 and thrombocytes 89,000.

On May 24, our clinic recommended CoD Tea to Dr. Apostolos Georgopoulos, chief of the chemotherapy and microbiology section of the Vienna University clinic. Ruth was released and her father assumed responsibility for CoD treatment.

On May 30, Ruth was again admitted to the hospital with a fever of 39°C (104°F). Blood levels: leukocytes 14,000, thrombocytes 49,000. This visit was also to serve as preparation for a bone marrow transplant. On June 4, 1995, Ruth was again released from the hospital. She had a minimal fever (37.8 and 37.3°C), and slept quietly. On June 8, she developed a fever again. Her doctor ordered a thrombocyte infusion.

On June 12, Ruth stopped CoD Tea treatments as part of her preparation for a bone marrow transplant. On July 5, a round of chemotherapy began in order to weaken Ruth's immune system so her body would not reject the transplanted bone marrow. Doctors treated her persistent fever with cortisone.

Suddenly, Ruth's condition deteriorated significantly. Blood levels: leukocytes 650, thrombocytes 4,000. On July 17, she was transferred to the intensive care unit with fluid in her lungs and chest cavity. A puncturing of the lung brought some relief.

On July 19, results of lung tests were nearly normal, and the heart had clearly improved. Her blood levels were alarming, however: leukocytes 500 (just a fraction of that of a healthy person); and thrombocytes 4,000 (merely an eighth of normal levels).

On July 24, in view of her life-threatening blood levels, she was again started on CoD Tea. Her blood levels improved slightly: leukocytes 880; thrombocytes 27,000.

By the next day, Ruth's condition had improved considerably. The blood tests showed some promising results: leukocytes 1,350; thrombocytes 46,000.

This trend continued on the next day. On July 28, Ruth was again released from the hospital. Her blood levels were normal: leukocytes 10,000, thrombocytes 280,000.

On July 28, a glowing Ruth came with her parents to visit me in my animal clinic. She played for hours with my cat, Doktor Doc. Her doctors had spoken of a miracle. Normally the blood levels of a transplant patient will take about six weeks to return to normal. For Ruth, the process had taken eight days.

Roland, age 4

Equally dramatic was the case of four-year-old Roland in Budapest. On May 12, 1996, I received a call from his father.

"My son's life is in danger. He's been diagnosed with cancer of the lymph nodes. He had a tumor in his ear, which was removed, but now there's a problem with his kidney. I'm desperate, and recently heard about your rainforest tea. Please help me. My son must live."

Istvan B. was not satisfied until I agreed to come to Budapest and meet him.

Three hours later, I sat across from Istvan B. in an outdoor cafe, and later that very night, Professor Georgopoulos and Dr. Balaun were consulting on the best treatment for Roland. Both recommended a course of chemotherapy concurrently with CoD Tea. They started immediately, the chemotherapy lasted from May 13 to May 18, 1996. Naturally, Roland's condition worsened during the chemotherapy.

On May 17, I went to pay a visit to Roland at the Budapest Pediatric Clinic. His body had reacted to the chemotherapy in the usual way. I understood the worries of parents who are expecting an inevitable catastrophe for their child. I tried to give them courage; after consulting with Roland's doctor, I was convinced that his abilities along with the rainforest tea would improve Roland's test results very quickly. Very often in the past year I had witnessed how resilient children can be. Still, an infection which had begun in Roland's mouth worsened as the chemotherapy progressed. He could barely drink anything, and did not want to eat. The sorrowful sight of their son devastated his parents more than Roland's catastrophic blood test results.

On May 27, Roland came down with a viral infection. He had a high fever and strong cough. But then on May 28, his blood levels improved dramatically, much as they had with Ruth.

On June 3, Roland's father got a call from the doctor, who told him that Roland's blood levels were completely normal. He had no more fever, and could return home. Only the infection in his mouth had not gone away. Since then, Roland has returned to kindergarten. He still takes the rainforest tea, his parents watch his diet, and they have never had cause to look at him with sad, pitying eyes as they had in May.

On December 20, 1996, I visited Roland in Budapest in his parents' apartment. We played "Indians" for almost two hours. This was my most wonderful Christmas present ever. His father proudly showed me Roland's latest test results—all of which were absolutely negative.

Caroline N., age 44

The case of Caroline N. is one in which I would by no means describe the patient as "nearly cured," as I might in the cases of both Roland and Ruth. For this reason, her case is more typical of others encountered in our experience with CoD Tea.

Ms. N. is forty-four years old. In September 1995 she was diagnosed with intestinal cancer. She decided against both surgery and chemotherapy.

On November 11 her doctor examined her and wrote the following report: "Compared with the last test results, I've determined a clear progression of tumor growth. The last CAT scan indicated that a tumor had spread in the intestine and had also become visible on the outer part of the vagina. Tumor growth has advanced considerably since the last examination, and at present is beginning to spread to the genital area, and there are even clear traces on the outer genitalia."

After this devastating report, Ms. N. learned of our Cancer Information Center in Budapest. She asked for help and wanted to try CoD Tea treatments, but she was worried about the cost. We agreed to provide her with tea at no cost.

Naturally, the big question was how we were going to pay for the tea, the airfreight costs (the plants had to be shipped by airfreight in order to guarantee freshness), lab tests, examination costs, and on and on.

What happened was that our research biochemists volunteered their time and skills in order to keep the project going.

In order to pay our Indian harvesters and transporters, I applied for several government and private grants, and when this turned out not to be enough, I applied for a loan, using my animal clinic as collateral. Naturally we would eventually be marketing the rainforest tea. Even today I still know that the great majority of terminally ill patients who have been working with us could never afford the costs of our tea if we ever tried to recover our costs and turn a profit.Thus I requested of our backers that we charge our patients based on their ability to pay. I thought that such a policy would appear neither too unrealistic nor too patronizing. I saw it as an obligation. I did not know who should or would take the responsibility when some of our patients suddenly had to give up taking the tea because they couldn't afford it. (Incidentally, most negotiations with potential business partners have fallen through because of this very point.)

But back to Caroline N. I would characterize the trajectory of her illness after taking CoD Tea as typical. Eight weeks after she began taking the tea, she returned for another examination and the same doctor, Dr. Gyorgy Bindics, made the following report:

"Contrast exam of the pelvis on January 1, 1996. On comparison with the previous tests on November 16, 1995, there has been an unusually clear and significant regression of the tumor.

"At present there seems to be just a light, uneven thickening of the rectum which shows the presence of a tumor. There are no indications that the tumor is spreading to the genital region. There are no indications of swollen lymph nodes."

I have never met Caroline N. personally, but received a copy of these reports from her, which she sent me along with a letter of thanks. In her letter she told me that she feels healthy, and that she started working again on February 1, 1996.

The CoD Tea and Nutrition System

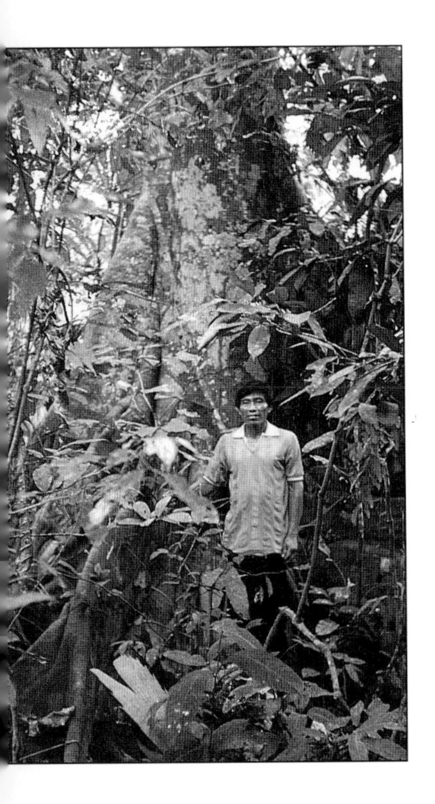

Collectors can determine which plants can be found in certain places with astonishing accuracy. They look for the amount of light, distance from riverbanks, and the types of plants in a given area.

Our positive results have indicated to me that in the last three years we've been on the right track in fine-tuning dosages and in developing an accompanying diet that will enhance the benefits of CoD Tea. Seven hundred forty-seven patients who had given up hope, and whose doctors had given them only months to live, began CoD treatment between November 1993 and March 1994. As of December 1995 seventy-five have died.

From all the data I've gathered over the years, I've determined that the CoD Tea and nutrition system works best for cancer patients who are resistant to or undergoing additional chemotherapy. According to Dr. Judah Folkman, the best time for surgery is 2–3 months after beginning the CoD Tea and nutrition system (with or without chemotherapy), when the size of the tumor has largely decreased. When tea treatment is initiated at this terminal stage IV phase of the illness, a patient normally shows a remarkable improvement within eight to ten weeks.

After many years of clinical experience, Dr. Folkman has come to the conclusion that the primary tumor should be removed in any case, as it presents an incalculable risk to the patient. Nevertheless, most patients who have undergone treatment with CoD Tea and have decided against surgery have stuck with their decision. Unfortunately, our observations have not been going on for a sufficient length of time to determine whether these cases have had positive results or not. Speaking for myself, I can only say that if I were faced with a similar situation, I would most certainly follow Dr. Folkman's advice.

In any case, it is essential that each patient seeks the advice of his or her doctor or specialist. In no case should CoD treatment be carried out without the supervision and advice of a medical professional.

Notwithstanding the many positive experiences, I would

never be so bold as to suggest that the CoD system is a cure for cancer. I do believe, however, that in most cases, many of which were thought to be hopeless, patients who took CoD Tea were able to lead a dignified and independent life, free of pain.

The reduction of pain allows the patient to sleep, which often helps stimulate the appetite. As a result, many patients gain a few pounds, which in turn results in added strength and energy. Many have been able to do some light work around the house or indulge in a hobby, as long as it's not a strenuous sport.

The CoD Tea treatment consists of the CoD herbal tea—a mixture of mainly tropical plants—as well as green tea and sage tea.

Preparing CoD Tea

CoD Rainforest Tea is simple to prepare, although we've heard many patients complain, "Why don't you have any capsules or tablets or drops? If you did, I could be much more independent in my free time, or when I'm traveling."

I must admit that such complaints actually make me profoundly happy. To think that these patients have been afflicted with a fatal disease yet, within a few weeks, they have progressed from hopeless cases concerned with sheer survival to a point where they can go out to a restaurant or even take a trip!

Preparing CoD Tea is quite simple. These directions follow the shaman's recipe to the letter:

1. Place and mix 3 to 20 grams (1 tsp. to 2–3 tbsp.) of tea in an enamel pot filled with 1/2 liter of water.
2. Let it sit for 12 hours.
3. Add 1 liter of water and boil for 30 minutes over low heat.
4. Let cool, and top off with water to the 1 1/2-liter mark.

It is not an art to prepare CoD Tea in a way that will have optimal results in conjunction with the accompanying diet. It is more difficult to follow the diet, which is very strict. But the radical, wise changes in lifestyle and diet, together with the recommended physical and psychological exercises, are essential for the preservation of one's health. The rainforest tea is no wonder drug. It can relieve severe internal disturbances, but not if one continues to smoke, eat without limitations, consume alcohol, and not take care of one's body and soul. One must bring self-discipline to the healing of one's body, to activate one's own protective force and healing energy. Nothing can supplement this.

The following recommendations should be helpful for the mastering of these tasks.

Diet and Lifestyle Recommendations

The CoD diet is no weight-loss plan. It was designed to support the human convalescence process for those recovering from a serious illness or operation, and who want to begin to slowly rebuild their strength. It contains several foods which are meant to stimulate the appetite.

For these reasons, healthy or overweight people should not ignore this section, but should use the guidelines presented here as preventive measures for organic illness with irreversible consequences, or to find out if some kind of poisoning might be causing discomfort.

This diet is based on the knowledge and experience humanity has accumulated—for better and worse—over the millennia, and forgotten or repressed in our modern age of excess. If you are tempted by the eating habits and delicacies characteristic of this age, you will no doubt find that our diet requires a major adjustment. Anyone, however, who has even applied some sound principles to their eating habits will find that our diet requires only a few minor changes.

The original aim of this diet was to help clear the body of toxins. When we look at the diets of "primitive" societies, we notice that most of their side dishes, desserts, or between-meal snacks are usually foods which enhance the functions of the liver, kidneys, spleen, or colon.

Regardless of how primitive people live their lives, they all have this in common: their lifestyle is conducive to getting out in the fresh air. We, on the other hand, have developed a society and a way of life which guarantee that we have an almost constant deficit of oxygen, even though oxygen is the most essential source of nutrition for our cells. Spending some time out in the fresh air is not just essential for staying slim and in shape, it's essential for staying healthy.

Perhaps it would be easier to devote time to being active in the fresh air if we look at such activities, along with breathing exercises, as ways to regenerate and recuperate our body's cells. Additional oxygen refortifies the cells for their continual battle against toxins, viruses, and pathogenic cells.

Whether you are working or reading, watching TV or sleeping, billions of cells are constantly on the alert and ready to pounce on invaders and unwanted guests (cancer cells among them). Unfortunately, there is no early warning system that can trip some sort of alarm when healthy cells are in danger of losing the battle. I would recommend that anyone go for a checkup about six to eight months after any period of great physical or psychic stress. For example: persistent grief or sense of loss after losing a loved one (through either death or divorce), jaundice, persistent metabolic disturbance, or chronic cough. I would also recommend a radical, and immediate (or gradual, when appropriate) change in the diet as follows:

Caloric intake:

Adjust according to appetite, but stop before you feel full. Stick to a high-fiber, low-calorie diet. Total caloric intake will vary with each individual case, depending on your metabolism, activity, height, and weight. Please consult with your physician to decide what is right for you.

Meals:

Divide caloric intake among five meals:

Breakfast (approximately 25% of the daily caloric intake)
Morning snack (about 15%)
Lunch (about 30%)
Afternoon snack (about 15%)
Dinner (about 15%)

Preparation:

Food should be mostly raw, unprocessed, whole foods, boiled or steamed only. Start meals with raw vegetables and seeds. Prepare only as much as you will eat for each meal. Everything should be freshly prepared (no leftovers).

Vegetables, salad, fruits:

These should form the backbone of your diet. Use organic fruits and vegetables whenever possible.

Protein:

A maximum of 10 percent of your intake of protein should come from animal protein. The majority will be from plant sources, predominately soybeans, miso, or tempeh.

Fats and oils:

Minimal amounts of fats and oils, exclusively from plant sources, with a variety of polyunsaturated fatty acids, like flaxseed and olive oil (never heat flaxseed oil).

Carbohydrates:

Mostly rice (brown rice), whole-grain products—such as bread, baked goods, or pasta and potatoes.

Dairy products:

Only skim milk products, cottage cheese, yogurt, and very little cream, goat, and sheep cheese.

Sweeteners, salt, and spices:

Use only honey as a sweetener, and only sea salt and fresh herbs for spices. Use as little salt as possible.

Liquids (beverages):

CoD Tea, green tea, sage tea, mineral water (uncarbonated), freshly squeezed organic fruit and vegetable juices, rice and soy drinks. Avoid coffee and alcohol.

Summary

Food:

Ninety percent vegetables, fruits, soybeans, rice and whole grains. Ten percent animal protein—fish or poultry.

Beverages:

At least 3 to 4 liters of fluids daily. Preferably CoD Tea ($1\frac{1}{2}$ liters), sage tea ($\frac{1}{8}$ liter, 5 minutes before meals), green tea ($\frac{1}{4}$–$\frac{1}{2}$ liter, after meals), lemon juice, or freshly pressed carrot, apple, beet, artichoke, dandelion, milkthistle, orange, or grape juice, or herbal tea.

Herbs:

Use only fresh herbs, such as chives, parsley, dill, basil, marjoram, taragon, mint, oregano, thyme, sage, cress, lemon grass, etc.

Avoid herb mixtures containing salt, such as grilling or barbecue preparations, lemon pepper, Worcestershire sauce, taste additives.

Eggs:
Maximum of 3 boiled egg *yolks* per week. Avoid omelets and scrambled eggs.

Things to avoid:
Bacon, sausage, beef and beef products, pork and pork products, anything roasted, fried, smoked, pickled, salted, or grilled.

Alcohol, nicotine, coffee, sharp or synthetic spices, white flour, sugar, chocolate, cakes, sweets, butter, margarine, diet spreads, low-fat margarine.

Recommended:
High-fiber, low-fat intake. Concentrate on soybean products (miso, tofu, tempeh), Nori, broccoli, cauliflower, garlic, onions, tomatoes, white cabbage, artichokes, potatoes, brussels sprouts, cabbage, lettuce, asparagus.

Switch to whole foods (muesli, whole wheat and rye, oats, barley, wheat germ, etc.). Mix 1 teaspoon of flaxseed oil with 6 teaspoons of low-fat cottage cheese.

Eat a little bit of everything I've recommended, and be sure each meal is varied.

The last meal of the day should be approximately three hours before bedtime.

Give yourself a rubdown twice a day with a towel dipped in hot water with a little bit of peppermint oil.

Change your lifestyle! Alternate hot and cold showers. Strengthen your psyche, think positively, and do relaxation exercises, yoga, or visualization exercises. Run or swim three times daily for fifteen minutes. Do breathing exercises. Take a deep breath through the nose, hold the air in for a count of five, and breath out very slowly through the mouth. Repeat three times daily, about ten minutes each time. In this way you are activating the self-healing forces of your body and your soul. Enjoy your hobbies, enjoy your life!

Suggested Menus

Breakfast	Morning snack	Lunch	Afternoon snack	Dinner
an apple, apple juice or carrot juice	tomatoes	miso soup, green beans with boiled chicken or fish, bananas	yogurt with fruit, beet juice	vegetable salad with boiled tempeh
cottage cheese with kefir, rye bread, artichoke juice	apple	vegetable soup with miso, squash, white cabbage, egg, fruit	tomatoes, dandelion juice	steamed green beans with tofu
whole grain toast with honey, beet juice	grapes, apple juice, and carrot juice	miso soup, steamed fish with rice and zucchini, fruit with honey, lemon juice	waldorf salad, milk thistle juice	potato with cottage cheese and dandelion salad
black bread with cottage cheese, artichoke juice	yogurt with sliced bananas	rice soup, steamed tofu with millet, carrots with lemon juice	whole grain roll with goat cheese, dandelion juice	spinach with turkey, fruit salad

Patient Reports

I'd like to tell you about this book's beginnings. In the autumn of 1994 I was at an art exhibit, and by chance I ran into a publisher friend of mine whom I hadn't seen in months. Several years before, I had shown him photos I had taken while sailing around the Greek islands in the Aegean Sea. From my passion for photography, he whipped together a nicely illustrated and successful book on the life of the Greek islands.

When we met at the exhibit he was naturally curious to know what I had been up to. In between stuffing myself with free sandwiches and wine, I told him of my experiences in the rainforest and of our first clinical successes using rainforest tea. He listened carefully, asked a few questions, and said, just as he had several years earlier when he looked at my pictures of Greece, "We've got to make this into a book."

"No way. I have absolutely no time. First, I'm doing this research right now, which is hard enough. Then I still have the clinic. Besides that, I'm trying to organize a harvesting, transportation, and distribution system with the Indians in South America. And if that's not enough, I've been in contact with another doctor from China. The Chinese also have a rich botanical tradition which goes back thousands of years. Their expertise has made it so I don't have to reinvent the wheel for the third or fourth time."

I'm not sure if it was due to wine or my memory of how much fun it had been doing the Greece book, but I ended up agreeing to do another one after all.

As he had promised, the publisher sent me someone to assist me in putting a manuscript together. He was the Viennese journalist Werner Stanzl, and since our first meeting I've spent many days and nights working with him. I have never, not even for one second, felt that his job has been to make this work any easier for me. Quite the contrary, most of the time I've been convinced that he's gone out of his way to make the whole project more difficult. An English colleague has accurately described him as "a pain in the neck," but I can think of several other phrases that come to mind.

I had no idea of the significance of his words on our first meeting, "Herr Doctor, I will always be asking the same questions: Who, Where, When, What, and Why? These are the five Ws of journalism, the tools of our trade."

First, I gave Stanzl a quick rundown of our successes. At that time, about twelve hundred terminally ill patients were taking our tea. Of those who were strictly following the prescribed diet, approximately 80 percent were doing significantly better. They were not in pain, could sleep without difficulty, and could eat and manage light work.

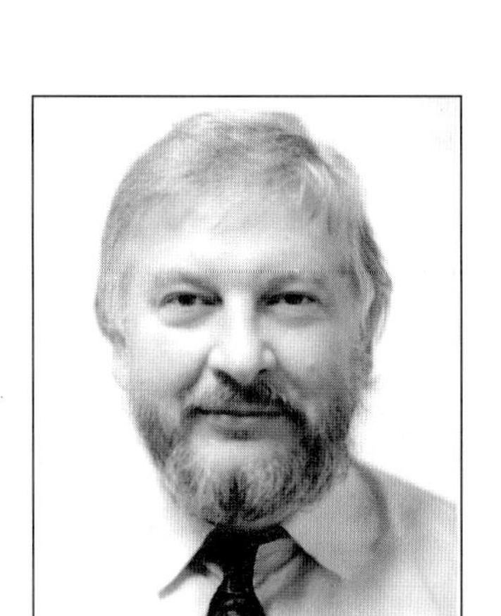

Journalist Werner Stanzl

After I had given this information, I asked, "So, what do you think?"

"Well, if you had told me that 10 percent of your patients had improved, I would have been more interested."

I should have left the room. Stanzl noticed my annoyance, and backtracked, "But I don't really see a problem. Certainly you've got twelve hundred names and addresses (He really didn't even believe the number!), so I suggest that I choose ten names at random, and pay them a visit."

On the way home, I passed my bookstore again. As it happened, there were several books in the display window on miracle cures and healers. It was clear that I would never bring one of these books home with me, to say nothing of reading them or even taking them the least bit seriously. I resolved to do my best to fulfill Stanzl's demands for a successful collaboration.

The next day, I had my secretary contact cooperating doctors and clinics in Hungary, where most of our patients were located, so they could secure permission from the patients, agreeing to an interview with Stanzl.

After that, I called Stanzl and invited him to the clinic. I handed him a folder with patient consent forms, giving Stanzl permission to interview them. Stanzl was astonished and, in no time, began sniffing around.

A Journalist on the Trail

By Werner Stanzl

In the fall of 1995 I received a call from a publisher friend of mine. He asked me to contact Dr. Thomas David with the intention of publishing a book on his research. Dr. David was a very busy man, and perhaps I could be of some help to him. My friend vouched for his credibility.

There are any number of books on the market on the all-too-well-known theme of miracle healers, and there have always been unscrupulous charlatans to prey upon the desperation of terminally ill patients for profit. I entered into this project with great skepticism, and thought I knew how it was going to turn out.

I had already met Dr. David on one occasion. It was at a party, and I remember that the gossip of the day had been about a head surgeon at a Viennese hospital who had accidentally inserted a pacemaker in the wrong patient. At this party, Dr. David staunchly defended the surgeon. He said earnestly that it could happen to anyone, and that the man happened to be a first-rate surgeon who had earned the respect of his colleagues.

My response was, "I'm sure he earns a lot."

Later, after examining the case more carefully, I determined that the surgeon really was innocent, but my opinion of Dr. David had not improved one iota.

I wanted to quickly and painlessly get this project out of the way. Before I could get bogged down in details, I wanted to interview some patients. I was certain I would never hear from Dr. David again, and that would be the end of it.

Much to my surprise, he called me two or three weeks after our first meeting and invited me to his clinic to get some patient addresses. In his office, without saying a word, he gave me a giant box filled with consent letters from patients in his Budapest clinic. I chose two envelopes at random.

"These are nearly all Hungarian addresses," I said, astounded.

"Well, it was a lot of work, and since work is cheaper in Hungary, I had my people there take care of it."

A Visit to Erika T.

One address stood out. It was from Erika T., in Tuscany. What was unusual was that she was diagnosed not with cancer, but with AIDS. Dr. David explained to me that cats who had been infected with AIDS and given CoD Tea had shown a remarkable recovery in immune response. This had resulted in a stabilization or increase of the T-lymphocyte count, and no active symptoms. Dr. David had supplied the tea to some AIDS patients who had requested it, usually at no cost.

What's a poor journalist to do? It was autumn, and time for the grape harvest in Tuscany, so I decided to mix business with pleasure and visit Erika.

She told me that she had come to Tuscany from Hungary to work as a receptionist in a hotel. She fell in love with a young Italian who told her before their first intimate encounter that he was HIV positive. Their trust in the safety of condoms was so great that they were married.

Soon it became clear that their trust in the condom was misplaced. One horrific day in 1993, Erika learned the terrifying news that she was HIV positive.

"Although I had lost some of my fear of AIDS because of my experience with my husband, I was still desperate. I wanted to go back to Budapest and die. Three days later, I was lying in my mother's arms. She had heard of some tea from South America. A friend who had had lung cancer had tried it, and it had done wonders.

"Through a very roundabout way, we got the address of a Cancer Information Center in Budapest. I took all the money I had been saving and went there to get some of the tea. They made me feel very welcome, and told me I wouldn't have to pay anything. They also told me I'd have to follow a strict diet. I asked if I could give some to my husband as well. They said sure, but warned me that it certainly wouldn't be able to cure AIDS. The most it could do was minimize any outbreaks. 'For years?' I asked them. 'Maybe,' they said."

Erika returned to Italy to tell her husband about the tea. He had been infected in 1990, and had recently begun showing signs that full-blown AIDS was making an appearance. His knees were swollen, and he had had the flu for months.

"About six weeks after he started taking the tea, my husband had no more symptoms. As for me, I have yet to have any symptoms at all. I wouldn't even know I was sick if the doctors hadn't told me."

I wanted her to tell me again. "How much did they charge you for this tea?"

"Nothing. I get a delivery once a year. They only asked that we keep them informed of our progress, which I do."

I wished Erika well and went on my way. My trip had been

unproductive. Many HIV patients can lead normal lives for years after becoming infected, without showing any signs of illness. My visit to Erika's doctor confirmed that there were no signs of an outbreak in Erika's case, but, given the time that she had been diagnosed as HIV positive, this was nothing unusual. It was the same for her husband. The symptoms he had had a few months before could have been caused by anything. His swollen knee could have been simply related to physical exertion. "He's a mason," said the doctor, "and when he spends his days on the job, carting wheelbarrows full of cement, it can put a real stress on his knee. On top of that, Italy was hit by a major flu epidemic recently. Thousands came down with it, and my office was full through most of the summer."

I asked the doctor his opinion of the tea, and let him know that I was skeptical; I didn't want to be laughed out of his office.

But he said, "Don't underestimate nature. If your Dr. David had claimed that some tea or a new diet could *cure* cancer, I would be skeptical, and if he charged a thousand lire for a package of his tea, I would have taken him for a charlatan. But when he says that the tea can help *improve* the patient's quality of life, and he *gives* it away, if I were in your place, I'd do my homework too, and check the facts. We have our own herbs here in Tuscany. I've had terminally ill patients under constant and severe pain. Instead of doping them up, I prefer to give them an herbal tincture. At least they can sleep without losing control of their senses.

"Do you know how much it means for a terminal patient to be able to sleep? Don't say 'yes,' because I can tell you right now that you have no idea. I've heard a few things about mistletoe tea. I don't know anything substantive about it, so I'm hesitant to give any specifics. But you have names and addresses of patients. I'd suggest you don't waste any time, and look them up and ask them. Even if your visit with Erika hasn't been all that useful."

So I went on to Budapest. There I learned that many of the patients had absolutely no objections to my using their names and addresses. Josef Marcali Kiss, a painter, explained, "Look, anyone who has had cancer of the lymph nodes, as I have, is eager to speak with others with the same condition who have taken the tea. If anyone writes to me, I'd be glad to give them an answer. And if I get letters from more than a hundred, I'll just photocopy a letter and send it. I'm glad to do anything I can to help. I really think you should use my name and address."

Other patients were reluctant to give their names because they were hoping to return to work, and were afraid that public knowledge of such a serious illness could have serious consequences, such as a forced early retirement. Others did not want their relatives to find out about the seriousness of their illnesses. Among this last group, I learned to value the argument, "Can't do it . . . medical confidentiality!" But back to my list. Next on my list was Auguste O.

Auguste O.

Age 47

Lung cancer

Auguste first visited the Austrian-Hungarian Cancer Information Center in Budapest on July 6, 1995. She started taking the tea on July 8, 1995. On September 25, 1995, she wrote the following to the Cancer Information Center:

"As you know, I've been taking the tea since July 8. This is the only chance I have to keep on living and to be able to rest. I didn't want any more radiation therapy; it was making me horribly sick, and my tumor did not seem to be responding. At present I'm taking only your tea. My latest test results have shown that my tumor is at basically the same stage it was when I began taking the tea. According to my radiologist, it may have even receded slightly. Up to now, I am happy to report that I have experienced no side effects due to the tea."

Mrs. O. lives in a third-floor apartment not far from the venerable Hotel Gellert. When I first tried to visit her on the morning of October 12, 1995, no one was home.

She had no telephone, so I wasn't able to make an appointment before my visit. Her neighbor told me, however, that Mrs. O. liked to take a walk along the Danube every day. Evidently, she was doing quite well. According to her neighbor, Mrs. O. had had a cold in the spring, and had been coughing a lot at night ("You can hear everything through these thin walls!"), but that cleared up. I was lucky, the neighbor continued, to catch Mrs. O. in Budapest at all. She had just returned from a visit to her daughter in Australia. The neighbor asked me if I was a relative, and I answered with another question, and let her go on some more.

Evidently, she was not aware of Mrs. O.'s condition. I tried again in the afternoon, and Mrs. O. opened the door. Without exchanging more than a few words, I showed her a letter of introduction from the Cancer Information Center, and she gestured warmly for me to come in.

"Yes," she said, "I did have the flu this spring. At first I thought it had something to do with my cancer, but my radiologist at the hospital told me it was nothing to worry about. My tumor had not grown. In fact, it had gotten smaller since my last examination in January.

"I'm still taking the tea. At first, I thought it was disgusting, but I've gotten used to it. By the time I made my first visit to the cancer counseling center, I had already gotten used to the idea of dying. I wasn't afraid of dying anymore, but I was afraid of the pain. I'd heard so much about it. I only had one wish left in my life, and that was to pay one last visit to my daughter and my two-year-old granddaughter in Australia."

Mrs. O. brought out some photographs. "In August, I was able to fulfill my wish, and stayed for six weeks in Melbourne. It was wonderful! When my doctor first advised me to go ahead and go to Australia, I wasn't so sure. I didn't want to have to go to the hospital there, and have my daughter get stuck with the bill. I've always heard about how expensive medical care is in Australia. Actually, my neighbor does know about my cancer. She's the only one around here who knows. She's the only person I know who will take care of the funeral arrangements. She's promised me, and I feel relieved knowing it's all taken care of.

"My next exam is at the end of November. I don't think there's anything to be afraid of."

Mrs. O. pulled her left arm out of her sweater, and proudly showed me her Australian sunburn:

"Look at me. Now, my greatest wish is to be able to work again. I work at the Post Office, and I'll be able to return if my health allows. If it continues for much longer, I'll have to take an early retirement. I hope it doesn't come to that."

On December 2, 1995, I received a letter from Mrs. O. She explained that her exam went so well that she didn't need to return to the hospital until February 1996.

"The doctor wished me a Happy New Year, and I asked him, 'Will I survive it?'

"He said, 'If you continue like this, you'll experience the next millenium with no trouble, dear lady.' I think he was as happy as I was."

Paul M.

Age 46

Lung cancer, metastasis of the liver

First referred to the Cancer Information Center on April 9, 1995, Paul M. began the tea regimen and diet just days afterward.

Nearly one month later, on May 2, 1995, his wife wrote to the Cancer Center:

"I can hardly express my thanks to you for your advice and for the tea. This tea has given both my husband and our whole family hope that he'll be able to survive his difficult lung operation.

"I first learned that my husband had a metastasis in the liver on December 1, 1994. What was most astounding to us was how quickly the tea began to work. Before he started taking it, he often cried out from the pain, and neither he nor anyone in my family could even think about sleeping. But just a few days after he started taking the tea, the doctors reduced his morphine dosage. Now his doctor is prescribing tablets instead of injections. Both my husband and I are convinced that this improvement is due to the tea.

"Before he started on the diet and tea therapy, my husband suffered with severe back pain and had lost four kilograms. He often went for days without a bowel movement. But now, none of this is a problem. These days I find myself worried about his swollen knuckles, because I don't know what's causing the swelling."

Mr. M. and his family live in a small village south of Budapest. I sent them a letter announcing my upcoming visit, and several days later received an effusively friendly invitation from Mrs. M., in which she asked only that I not mention her husband's cancer in his presence.

When I arrived, Mr. M. was sitting on a bench in front of the house, enjoying a fine Indian-summer day.

His wife took us to the sitting room. She had just baked a Sacher torte, and there was hot coffee on the stove. Mr. M. cut into the torte enthusiastically, putting a smallish piece on his own plate. "I have to take it easy with baked goods," he said with a smile, and waited for his wife to continue.

"My husband is a bus driver, but he probably won't be going back to work anytime soon."

I could see a vegetable garden outside the window. Tomatoes were ripening on the vine, massive pumpkins lay on the loamy soil, waiting to be picked. "My husband does most of the garden work," said Mrs. M.

Mr. M. accompanied me to my car when it was time to go. "Don't think that I don't know why you're here. I found a slip of paper with a telephone number in my wife's things. I called, and when I found out it was the Cancer Center, I knew everything. My wife doesn't want me to know, so I try my best to humor her. If she knew that I knew, there'd be quite a scene. She absolutely hates it when I go through her things."

In January 1996 I received another letter from Mrs. M., in which she wrote that her husband was "doing well, very well."

Then her letter continued, "He seems to have given up hopes of ever driving again. I believe his rabbits are responsible. Before, he'd be satisfied with keeping three or four, but lately he's been hammering and sawing continually, building more cages. At present we have forty-six rabbits and, of course, more are on the way. I told him that we should sell a few, because we can't afford to feed them all.

"What amazes me most about him is how good he's been about sticking with the diet. Once, he even told me, 'You know, actually, I'm only eating what our rabbits eat. I've totally forgotten what meat tastes like.'

"We really have no other problems right now. By the way, he's known about his illness the whole time. And imagine how hard I've tried to keep it from him."

Josef Marcali Kiss

Age 60

Lymph cancer

As recently as August 1994, Josef Kiss had to be fed in the hospital. He wasn't able to walk, and could not even write his own name.

He began taking CoD Tea in December 1994. In January 1995 he wrote the following:

"I'm writing to ask you to help me continue my tea treatment.

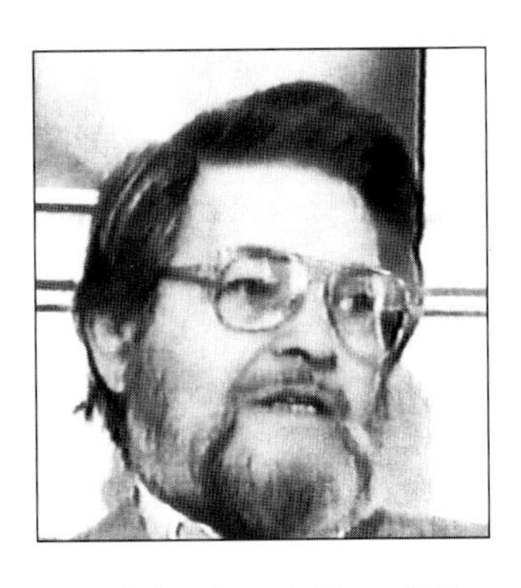

Painter Joseph Marcali Kiss: "I'm happy to share my experiences."

For four years, I've undergone chemotherapy treatments, only to have frequent relapses, and the tumors return. I've been weakened to the extent that it's unlikely I'll survive another stay in the hospital."

Here's an excerpt from Josef Kiss's hospital report in March 1995: "Patient has shown a marked improvement in physical and mental condition. He has started to gain weight. One lymph node shows a total remission, ten others show a 50 to 70 percent improvement, and another shows a 40 percent improvement. He is physically much stronger, and climbed the stairs to the second floor without any apparent difficulties."

Again, in September 1995, according to the report: "Three-week sailing trip on Lake Balaton. Patient is in outstanding physical and emotional condition."

Joseph Marcali Kiss lives in a pleasant neighborhood in the southwest of Budapest. The area is marked by gently sloping hills and many gardens. The focal point of Mr. Kiss's home is his painting studio, where he told me of his troubles, and of his unpleasant experiences with chemotherapy. He had just about given up hope when his daughter happened to hear about the Budapest Cancer Information Center, and about some tea that was supposed to have helped a lot of people. Mr. Kiss was eager to try anything that did not involve chemotherapy, and started to take the tea. The results of this treatment can be seen in the note he jotted down as an afterthought to his last letter to the Cancer Information Center: "I'm exercising for thirty minutes every day. Look out, I just might show you something."

He pushed aside the curtain that covered his studio wall. I saw paintings with menacing-looking black birds. I felt a distinct chill in the air.

"This is how my illness has influenced my painting. I haven't painted these consciously, I simply sat down and said to myself, 'so, paint some black birds.' I can only follow my muse, and this is where my muse had been leading me."

Here, he did an about-face, and said, "And here's what I paint today!" He pointed to another wall where there were pictures with white birds, soaring on the wind. He took one of the paintings off the wall, so I could look more closely. I saw several small figures standing in front of a silver-gray stage curtain. They seemed to be bowing and thanking an unseen audience. Some of the figures could have been clowns, while others had their arms extended gracefully upward, like ballet dancers soaking up an ovation after a rousing performance.

Mr. Kiss seemed as happy as a man could be, having passed the hardest test life has to offer.

"If you had one wish," I asked, "what would it be?"

He gushed, "Well, to tell you the truth, I did have a wish. I love to sail, and I have a small boat. If I'm out on Lake Balaton, it's pretty hard to make my tea, and I started to wonder how it would be if I could get it in a capsule or tablet. I wouldn't need to be near a stove every day."

In January 1996 Mr. Kiss wrote the following to the cancer center: "I'm constantly modifying my diet according to my lab test results, and what I can tolerate. Overall, I feel good, and my enthusiasm for work is satisfactory. I have no symptoms at present, and I have hopes for the future."

Again in March 1996: "On February 20, I went to my doctor for a follow-up visit. I had no symptoms or complaints. My lymph nodes have shown no change in these last wonderful months."

The last report from his physician, Dr. Schneider, reads, "liver has decreased in size by four centimeters. No evidence of further tumor growth. Patient's condition is stable."

Eleméméné Orban

Age 77

Cancer of the bladder

Mrs. Orban gives a strong first impression. She appears resolute, proud, and self-confident. Perhaps this is due, in part, to her habit of going (against both her diet and her doctor's orders) to a cafe in Budapest, and allowing herself to smoke one cigarette a week.

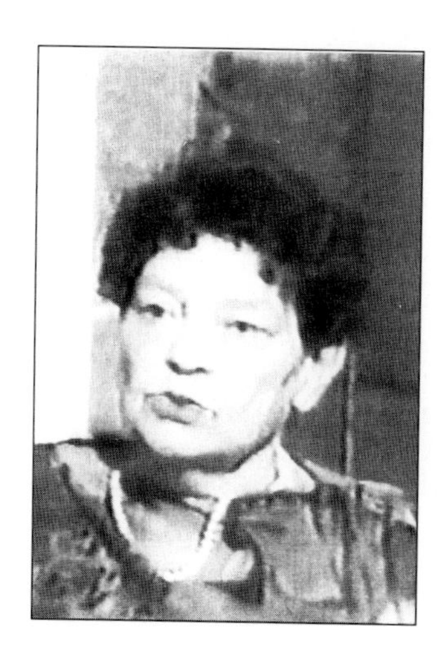

Elemerne Orban: she won her bet.

In August 1994 her doctor told her that she had a tumor the size of an egg on the wall of her bladder. He wanted to operate and remove it.

"Absolutely out of the question," she said.

She was all the more convinced since, a year and a half before, her brother had come to a "pathetic end" after having had an identical operation.

After she received the devastating news, she heard about a tea made from two plants. She tried it, but after a few weeks she only felt worse. In October 1994 she gave in to her doctor's pleas and consented to have the tumor removed by laser in a series of operations. She would still not consent to chemotherapy or radiation therapy.

In November, while she was in Austria, she had heard about the Budapest Cancer Information Center and CoD Tea. She began taking the tea in November.

"After only four weeks I felt significantly better. I sent my daughter to the hospital, to tell my doctor that I did not want him operating on me anymore. My daughter told me that my doctor had bet me a bottle of champagne that I'd be back for my next operation within three months.

"I continued drinking the tea, and stuck with the diet, and in January of '95 returned for a follow-up exam. I felt wonderful, especially when my doctor called me into his office, and said, 'You win. The latest X ray shows no sign of your tumor.' Afterward, I treated myself to some champagne. It was the best I've ever tasted, even though it was only the cheap Hungarian stuff."

In an envelope I had fished out of the box in Dr. David's office, I found the following lab report: "January 11, 1995. Urine test normal, blood test negative, CEA (carcino-embryonic antigen) levels have returned to normal, we have only detected a scar from the tumor on the bladder wall." A subsequent examination on May 12, 1995, was nearly identical, except for the conclusion: "Patient is in outstanding physical and mental condition."

I asked Mrs. Orban how she liked the taste of the tea.

"Even bad white wine tastes better," she complained.

"And the diet?"

"I treat myself to a cigarette every now and then, but otherwise, I've been pretty good."

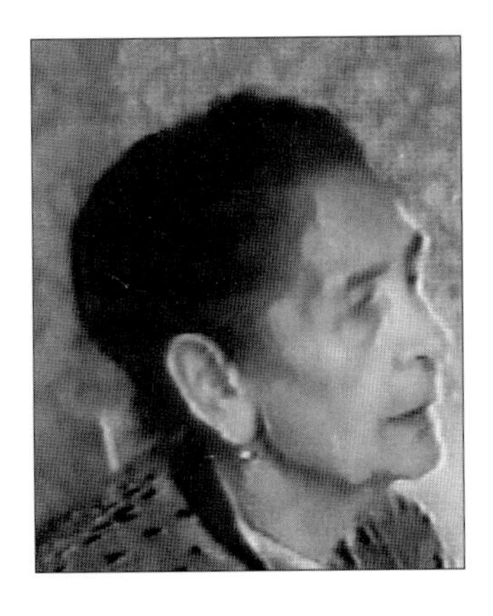

Nurse Elisabeth, 79: improved immune response.

The Nurse

My next interview took me to a seventy-nine-year-old woman who lived just outside of Budapest. She had been diagnosed with pancreatic cancer. She asked me not to use her name because she was in no condition to respond to anyone who might try to contact her.

She had been a nurse in the operating room. Before she had her pancreas removed, her doctor warned her that only two out of ten patients survive the procedure. She began tea treatment one month after the operation. Due to her age, chemotherapy was considered out of the question.

By May 1995 her condition had improved so much that she could continue her favorite summertime hobby. She proudly showed me shelves filled with canned strawberries, rhubarb, cherries, apricots, and pickles. In the corner of her basement sat a barrel of fermenting sauerkraut.

"Most of this is for my family," she said proudly, "but if my condition stays as it is now, I may eat some next year."

I went to visit her again on a Sunday in April 1996. She had just returned from church with her son and daughter-in-law. You could see absolutely no difference between her and other women her own age, except that she stood a bit more upright than some of the farmers. Her son confirmed that she was doing very well. In fact, she had had more difficulty recuperating from a gall bladder operation five years before.

As I was about to leave, she took me into her cellar again. "Remember my fruit? Take a jar of apricots. I have more than enough, and we're expecting a good harvest this year."

By now, I had little doubt that there really was something to Dr. David's rainforest tea. As luck would have it, on my return to Vienna, Dr. David held a report under my nose, which read:

"The results of our clinical tests clearly show that the application of CoD plant extract contributes to an increase in all functions measured. This in turn results in a beneficial in vivo effect on the granulocytes, and an improved immune response."

The renowned Dr. A. Georgopoulos of Vienna General Hospital had signed the report. I was impressed. Not just because of Dr. Georgopoulos's reputation, but the fact that he was a die-hard believer in the beneficial effects of chemotherapy, and was not one to take competition to scientific medicine lightly.

I could safely say that my investigation was over, but since Dr. David had enlisted the services of Dr. Judah Folkman, I decided to pay Folkman a visit to find out more about how CoD Tea actually works.

A Visit with Dr. Folkman

It wasn't easy to get an appointment to see Dr. Folkman. His secretary told me numerous times that he could not be disturbed. Finally, I was able to get his private fax number from the friend of a friend.

Writing to him was not easy. I thought hard about every single word. I wanted to spark his interest in the tea without having him think I was some kind of nut who had been taken in by a charlatan. In three weeks, I received an answer. He could meet me on July 9, 1996, between 9:00 and 10:30 A.M.

Folkman listened patiently, and then explained, "Let's assume that this tea works as you say it does. It's still impossible to say what it does without painstaking clinical trials. One thing we do know: there are substances found in nature which can hold metastases in check, and keep them from growing into full-blown tumors. Angiostatin was one substance that I discovered several years ago. In the time since, I've isolated thirteen other proteins which work similarly. Who knows, maybe we'll find two or even three hundred more. They might be found in plants or mammals or humans. We're going to be searching for a long time."

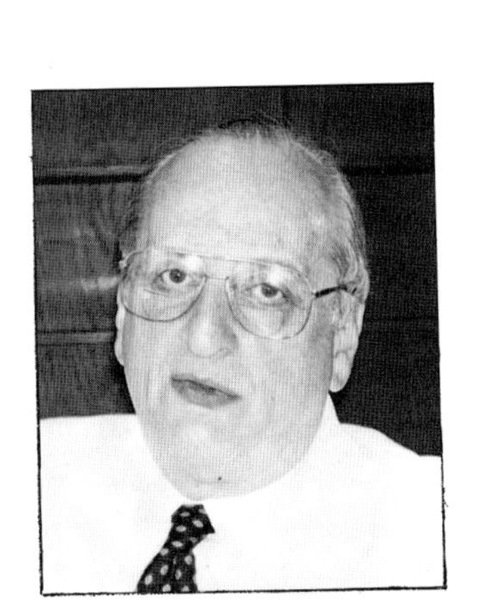

Dr. Judah Folkman of Harvard Medical School.

"So angiostatin is produced by the primary tumor to keep metastases in check. Have I understood that correctly?"

"Yes, that's right."

"Does that mean you can tell from a blood test that there is an active tumor in my body, even though I might not be aware of it?"

"Good question. Yes, theoretically, it's possible, but you'd never survive the test. I'd need about ten liters of blood to know for sure. If we took a small sample of blood and you tested negative for angiostatin, it wouldn't really tell us anything. I'm convinced that the next twenty years of research will provide us with a reliable early-warning system for cancer. Hopefully we'll be able to test just a miniscule amount of blood and know with some certainty. Think how complicated earlier forms of blood sugar tests or pregnancy tests used to be, and how long it would take before you had the results. Now it's all done in a matter of seconds. The hope is that this will be true for cancer testing as well. It would be a great help."

Naturally, I told him that, in my opinion as a layman, it was absurd that angiostatin wasn't being used as a medication. Unfortunately, there are many legal obstaces involved in putting a new drug on the market, and Dr. Folkman appeared—although reluctantly—to be trying his best to leap through the necessary bureaucratic hoops. I won't print his

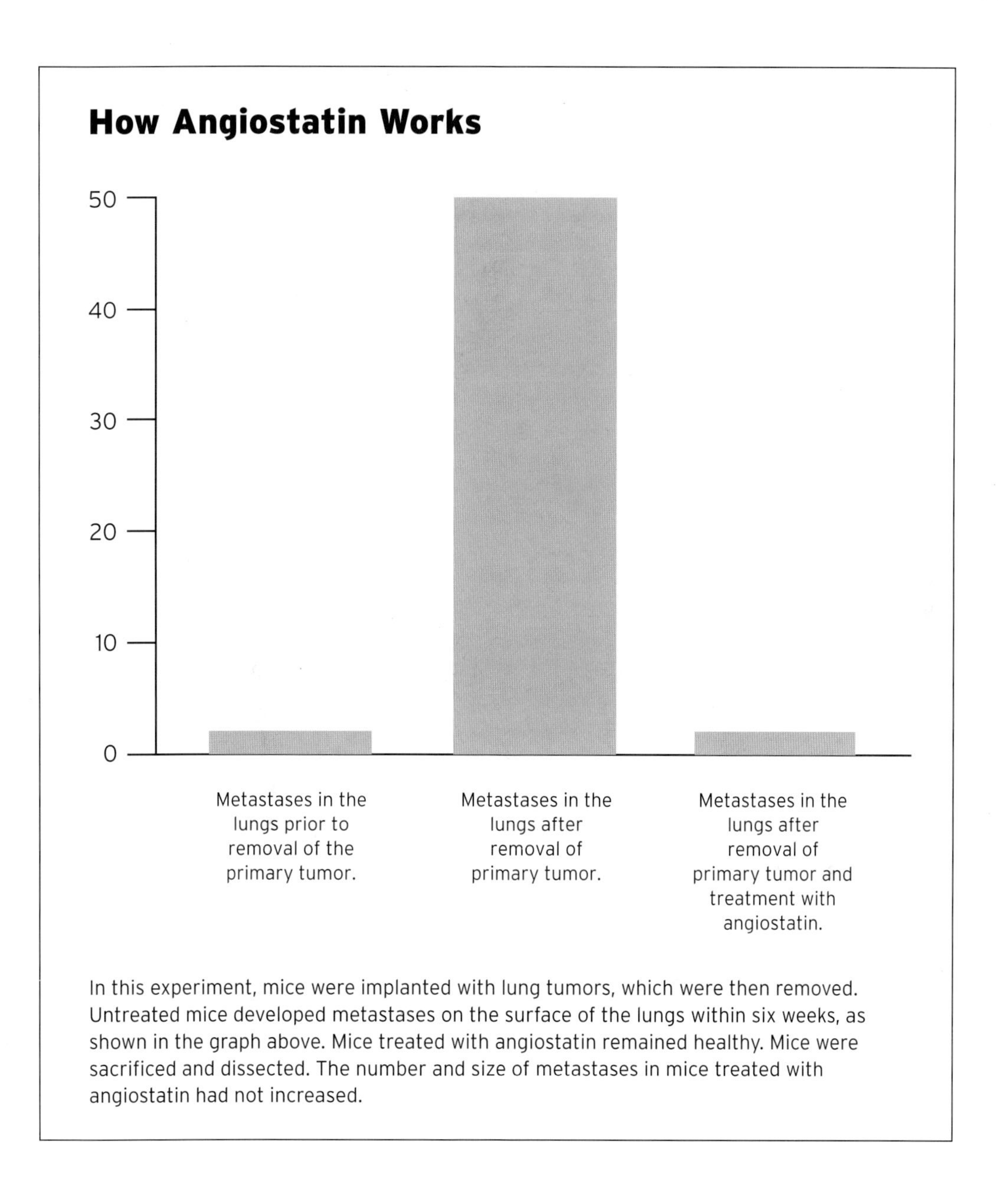

In this experiment, mice were implanted with lung tumors, which were then removed. Untreated mice developed metastases on the surface of the lungs within six weeks, as shown in the graph above. Mice treated with angiostatin remained healthy. Mice were sacrificed and dissected. The number and size of metastases in mice treated with angiostatin had not increased.

opinions concerning the red tape he's had to go through, but will only note that at this point our conversation had become confidential.

CoD Tea and Nutrition System in Use

When Werner Stanzl returned from Budapest, he was still not thoroughly convinced of the effects of CoD Tea. I noticed, however, that he seemed to have developed second thoughts about his heavy smoking habit, and was trying to cut down. If he noticed a burning sensation in his lungs, he'd ask me about the survival rates of lung cancer patients, and if he felt over-full after a large lunch, he'd ask me about stomach cancer.

"I know," he said, "it's all in my head. I once did a series with my partner on Sexually Transmitted Diseases. We had a very tight deadline, and we immersed ourselves so thoroughly in our subject that we began to imagine that we had contracted every one of them. They say that if you talk about fleas, you're bound to start scratching."

I mention all this because Stanzl had raised the question of using the tea as a preventive treatment. At the time, I was so involved in my research that I hadn't stopped to consider the question. I could only say, "Healthy Indians drink the tea as well. It's a kind of daily tonic for them. I have no idea if it can help prevent tumors in a healthy individual, and it would take several generations to test it properly. So I really don't know if it's useful in prevention or not. I only know that if you follow our diet, you'll stay healthy and the chances of contracting cancer will be minimal. Your diet and lifestyle affect your risk of cancer as much as they do with heart disease."

A study published by the World Health Organization determined that countries with a low frequency of heart attack (such as Japan and China) also have a low incidence of cancer. On the other hand, the report mentioned the United States, Germany, and Hungary as countries with very high rates of fatalities due to both heart disease and cancer.

So, if you stick to the prescribed diet, you reduce your risk of developing heart disease and cancer. I'm convinced that there isn't some wonder drug that would allow us to avoid the consequences of an unhealthy lifestyle. Such a drug would contradict the laws of nature, and if we have learned one thing in our age, it's this: we cannot contradict the laws of nature.

In this section, you will find reports from some terminal patients who have been kind enough to share their experiences with CoD Tea. These are just a sample selected from several hundred.

I didn't want to print them at first. Most of them are simply sincere thank-you letters, or the expressions of deeply felt relief, and should be taken as nothing more than that. But Stanzl thought we should print them.

"Any reader who is afflicted with lung cancer will certainly want to correspond with someone who has had experience with your treatment. I'm sure that many of your patients will be happy to share their experiences."

I wasn't totally convinced, but he did have a point. Certainly the exchange of experiences and information is important for anyone with a terminal illness. My institute in Vienna will gladly forward any correspondence we receive to any of the patients listed here.

Patients Share Their Experiences

All excerpts in the following section are from letters written by patients or their relatives and addressed to our Cancer Information Center in Budapest.

Dr. Irene A.
Born 1942
Diagnosed with breast cancer
She writes in February 1996: "I've been taking CoD Tea since November 11, 1995. My general condition has improved substantially, and my appetite has improved as well. My lymph edema has gotten smaller, and can now be massaged out. I'm also pleased to report that my rashes and itching have disappeared."

Mr. Laszlo A.
Born 1953
Diagnosed with a lung tumor
His wife reports in January 1996: "Since my husband has been taking your tea, he feels much better. He's stronger and has a good appetite. It seems to have a regenerating and stabilizing effect on his condition."

Ms. Stefanie B.
Born 1941
Diagnosed with breast cancer
She writes in January, 1996: "I've been taking your wonderful CoD Tea since November. Since then my condition has improved considerably. My appetite has improved and I have much more energy.

"Last fall, I needed help around the house, but now I can take care of myself.

"My face has a normal, healthy color again, and I believe that all of this is thanks to your rainforest tea."

Mr. Karl B.
Born 1925
Diagnosed with cancer of the liver

His wife writes in October 1995: "My husband has been taking your tea for only two weeks, and he's already feeling better. Before he started taking it, he was still bed-ridden, but since taking it, his appetite is back, and his mood has improved considerably."

Dr. Béla C.
Born 1926
Diagnosed with metastases of the liver

Dr. C. writes in November 1995: "After a difficult operation, I've been taking your tea for months with positive results."

In February 1996 he adds: "Thank you so much for your rainforest tea. My overall condition and my enthusiasm for work have been much stronger for several months. I'm not losing any more weight, and your diet hasn't increased my expenses at all."

Mr. Johann C.
Born 1967
Diagnosed with a brain tumor

He writes in October 1995: "Thank you for everything you've done for me. Your rainforest tea has been a major factor in my healing process."

Mr. Imre D.
Born 1946
Diagnosed with lung cancer

He writes in March 1996: "I want to thank you for helping me to fight this terrible illness, especially since out here in the provinces nobody cares about people with cancer. . . . I've been taking your rainforest tea since January 31. Since that time my general condition and my mood have improved. I'm strong enough to work again, and I can walk and even ride a bicycle. I'm sleeping much better and my appetite has returned. I'm trying to follow your diet, and I'm eating very well."

Mr. Enzo D.
Born 1942
Diagnosed with leukemia

"I've been taking your rainforest tea since the autumn of 1994. My condition has improved considerably since my last chemotherapy treatments. I'm back to my normal weight, and I feel fine. I even like the diet you've recommended."

Mr. Iván D.
Born 1933
Diagnosed with lung cancer

He writes in January 1996: "I thank you for your help, and pray to God that He will help you in your cause of helping and healing those with serious illnesses. I want to be healthy again; please help me."

Ms. Auguste E.
Born 1934
Diagnosed with breast cancer

She writes: "I can't believe what you've done for sick people. Of the several patients who had their operations around the same time I did, several have passed away. Unfortunately, they didn't discover your miracle rainforest tea. I am very thankful to have had the chance to take part in your research."

Mr. Béla F.
Born 1951
Diagnosed with lung cancer

He writes in December 1995: "My last examination showed essentially the same results as the previous exam. Most importantly, my tumor had not grown. Most of the others who were examined at the same time had experienced a deterioration of their condition and growth of their tumors. I've given your address to them, and hope you can supply them with tea free of charge."

Ms. Johanna F.
Born 1939
Diagnosed with breast cancer

She writes in February 1996: "I started taking your tea in June 1995. Since then, I have been feeling much stronger and my mood is positive. I feel your tea has helped me. pplease thank the professor who has made all this possible. With the help of this tea, I've been able to begin the healing process."

And again on March 12, 1996, she adds: "I thank you with all my heart for giving me the opportunity to take your tea. I've been staying on the diet you recommended. My test results are good, I feel much stronger, and my general condition has improved."

Mr. Stefan F.
Born 1958
Diagnosed with cancer of the testicles
He writes in February 1996: "After having taken your tea for one month, I feel much better than in the same period of time without having taken it. My spirits are much better, and I feel much stronger."

Mr. Paul F.
Born 1947
Diagnosed with lung cancer
He writes in December 1995: "I've been taking your tea for two months, and my condition has improved considerably. I don't get tired, and I don't need to take a break in the afternoon. I feel very lucky that my doctor had heard about you and gave me your address. My progress has made me very happy."

Ms. Leopoldine G.
Born 1932
Diagnosed with breast cancer
She writes in March 1995: "Shortly after I began taking your tea, I quickly experienced no longer having shortness of breath. I feel fine during the day, my appetite is healthy, and I'm sleeping well. . . . Up to now, the tea has had a very positive effect. I'm even able to take care of my grandchildren, which makes us all very happy."

Mr. Bruno G.
Born 1935
Diagnosed with lymphatic leukemia
He writes in February 1996: "I would like to respectfully express my heartfelt thanks to you for giving me the opportunity to try your tea. When I first heard of the rainforest tea just over one year ago, I was in a miserable state. Then your people made a program of the tea combined with a special diet. Since then I've been taking the tea and eating as directed and my test results, as well as my general condition, have improved. Please, on behalf of people like myself everywhere, I beg you not to give up the fight. I wish you continued success in your work."

Ms. Franziska G.
Born 1931
Diagnosed with breast cancer
She writes in March 1996: "I've been following your prescriptions for rainforest tea and a strict diet since January 10. I am happy to report that I currently have no symptoms. Sometimes I think that I'm totally cured. I am happy to be alive. At first, I started taking the tea just to humor my family. But now I feel I'm on the road to recovery and that my illness was just a bad dream. Sincerely, your strong healthy patient. . . ."

Ms. Ilona G.
Born 1933
Diagnosed with cancer of the lymph nodes
She writes in March 1996: "I've been taking your tea and following your diet since January 16, and I feel absolutely wonderful. My endurance is very good and my overall condition is good. I haven't been sick at all, even though my immune system had been devastated by my recent chemotherapy. I haven't even had a runny nose."

Ms. Irene H.
Born 1930
Diagnosed with breast cancer
Her daughter writes in January 1996: "My mother started taking your tea one year ago.

Since then, her appetite has returned and her mood has improved. She's gained two pounds. . . . Thank you very much for all that you've done for us. We really believe that this tea is helping her, and we hope that you will be able to continue sending it to us."

Irene writes in March 1996: "My latest blood tests were very encouraging, and lately I'm much calmer. My breasts are gone, but I try not to let it bother me, and I try to live as if nothing has happened. I always feel that I'm getting healthier and I can't give up hope. My blood pressure is normal and my appetite is quite good."

Ms. Andrea J.
Born 1948
Diagnosed with breast cancer

She writes in March 1995: "I've been taking the tea since January, and so far my experience has been very good. Since I started taking it, I feel much better overall, and my pain is not so intense. . . . I really believe the tea has been helping me for the last two months. My lab tests are promising."

Ms. Josephine K.
Born 1948
Diagnosed with breast cancer that had metastasized to the bone

On January 19, 1996 the isotope lab of the Komitats hospital reported: "The first picture was made on 1/10/1995. Compared with the previous examination, no progression can be detected.

"Opinion: metastasis cannot be found. She is doing fine. The blood count is normal. The oncology department says that the bone scan, chest X ray, abdominal ultra sound, and mammography are all negative.

"The tumor marker dropped significantly."

	January 9, 1995	January 20, 1996
CEA	1.37 ng/ml	1.3 ng/ml
CA 15-3	18.9 U/ml	6.2 U/ml
CA 125	15.9 U/ml	3.1 U/ml

Ms. Caroline K.
Born 1925
Diagnosed with lung and breast cancer

Her daughter writes in January 1995: "I believe your tea has been a great help to my mother. In the hospital, they had long given her up for dead. . . . The doctors told me it would be pointless to expect a recovery or to expect a miracle, but I've seen that that is not the case. She's doing much better, the edema on her foot is four centimeters smaller, and her appetite is much better."

Ms. Sandra K.
Born 1943
Diagnosed with intestinal cancer

She writes in December 1995: "You won't believe how much better I've felt since I began taking your tea. I feel more calm, relaxed, and secure, and I feel that this tea is protecting me. I don't obsess on my problems (like my husband's passing away, my eight recent operations, my hysterectomy). . . . It's been a great pleasure to drink your tea."

In March 1996 she writes again, "I can't thank you enough for giving me the opportunity to take your tea, and for sending it to me free. Thanks to you, I'm feeling so much better, and I feel that this tea is protecting me from all kinds of complaints. I'm not afraid anymore."

Mr. Karl L.
Born 1927
Diagnosed with cancer of the kidneys

His daughter writes in January 1996: "One month after my father started taking your tea his condition was visibly better. He goes for walks again, and is generally interested in life. In brief, I can say that clearly he is doing much better."

Karl L. writes in March 1996: "I would like to inform you that since I've been taking your tea, I've had no more fever. I'm getting better every day. I'm enjoying the diet very much, and have even gained three kilograms. Thank you for your generous help."

Ms. Ida L.
Born 1958
Diagnosed with encephalitis
She reports in June 1995: "I've been much better since I started taking your tea. Thanks to your diet and wonderful tea, I feel a thousand times better. It's clear that I'm improving and that the healing process has begun. My allergies have also disappeared without a trace this year."

Ms. Agnes M.
Born 1941
Diagnosed with lung and kidney cancer
She writes at the end of 1995: "Your tea has improved my condition and my skin has returned to its normal, healthy color. My appetite has improved, and I've gained three kilograms."

Ms. Rosa M.
Born 1917
Diagnosed with bone cancer
She writes in September 1995: "I've been feeling stronger every day since I started taking your tea, and I've been able to reduce the dosage of pain killers. I'm sleeping very well. Thank you for your help and generosity."

And in April 1996 she writes: "I'm making every effort to stick with your diet and avoid the foods that are off limits. Thanks to you and your tea, I'm not experiencing nearly as much pain as before, and I'm taking very small doses of pain killers. All this is thanks to your help."

Ms. Eugenie N.
Born 1935
Diagnosed with breast cancer
She writes in February 1996: "My doctor tells me that my blood tests are much better. I've modified my diet according to your instructions, otherwise I haven't changed my lifestyle all that much. I feel much better, and have more of an interest in life. I often go for walks, and my children have bought me a dog, which was quite a treat. I believe the tea has helped in my recovery."

Ms. Jenny P.
Born 1941
Diagnosed with cancer of the vulva
Her daughter writes in March 1995: "I'd like to thank you for providing my mother with your wonderful tea. . . . She began taking it in November 1994 and within a month her condition had improved significantly. Her mood has improved, which in itself is an accomplishment, and her appetite is much better. She even lectures me that I should watch what I eat and that I could learn a thing or two from your diet. Unfortunately, I have to settle for the company cafeteria."

Mr. Ian R.
Born 1931
Diagnosed with cancer of the kidney
He writes in the summer of 1995: "I started taking your tea in January 1995 and, since that time, my condition has improved considerably. I've even gone back up to my normal weight."

In February 1996 he writes: "My condition is even better. My weight has been stable for one year. At first, I had difficulty staying on the diet, but I've gradually gotten used to it. Currently, I'm visiting my five-year-old grandson, and I'm able to play with him and take walks. I'd like to thank you for giving me the opportunity to try your wonderful tea."

Ms. Josephine S.
Born 1942
Diagnosed with lung and breast cancer
She reports in March 1995: "This tea has saved my life. Before I started taking it, my condition had deteriorated so much that I had given up hope. I'm feeling mentally and physically better, the pain is not so strong, and I have hope again."

Mr. Erno S.
Born 1948
Diagnosed with intestinal cancer

He writes in November 1995: "I want to thank you for your generosity in sending me your tea free of charge. Since I started taking it, my appetite and general condition are much better, and I've been able to gain weight. . . . I hope that you will be able to continue supplying me with your wonderful tea."

Mr. Hans S.
Born 1932
Diagnosed with lung cancer

His stepson writes in November 1995: "The patient is in satisfactory condition. He's been taking the tea for eighteen months, and his appetite and test results are good."

Hans writes in February 1996: "Thank you so much for the tea you've sent me. I have a good appetite, both my general condition and my weight are stable. . . . My blood test in January was negative, and it's all because of your tea."

Ms. Tamara S.
Born 1942
Diagnosed with melanoma

She writes in February 1996: "I've been taking your tea regularly since March of last year. As I told you earlier, the tea seems to have a positive effect on inhibiting the growth of my melanoma. I am happy to report that I'm in good shape and, according to the latest lab results, my condition has stabilized. Thank you again for your wonderful work."

Ms. Michaela S.
Born 1932
Diagnosed with cancer of the larynx

She writes in February 1996: "I'm convinced that I've improved since I started taking your rainforest tea. My children are glad to see me smiling again. I hope you'll be able to continue supplying me with your tea."

Mr. Béla S.
Born 1928
Diagnosed with cancer of the lymph nodes

He writes in March 1996: "I am pleased to inform you that since I've been taking your tea, my condition has improved significantly. I'm not in as much pain, and my appetite has returned. In just a few months, I've gained five kilograms. My blood levels are much improved, and the growths on my lymph tumors have stopped growing. My doctor can't believe it."

Ms. Pauline S.
Born 1948
Diagnosed with breast cancer and bone cancer

Her daughter writes: Since my mother started taking your tea mixture, she has been doing much better. Her pain has diminished considerably. She lost quite a bit of hair during chemotherapy, and it has begun to grow back. She has no more nausea, even after chemotherapy treatments. Her appetite is back to normal, and she's gaining weight. . . . She doesn't tire as easily as she did before."

Ms. Karoline U.
Born 1938
Diagnosed with stomach cancer

She writes in January 1996: "Since I started taking your tea in November 1995, my condition has improved, and the tumor has stopped growing. My appetite is back to normal."

In February 1996 she writes again: "I've been following your diet very strictly, and my tumor has not advanced in the last two months. I'm meditating and praying. My strength and endurance are nearly back to normal. I'm up and around all day, and I am able to cook and iron and do light housework without tiring myself out. I feel I could do more vigorous work, but my doctor has advised me to take it easy. I've refrained from working in my garden, but I'm sure the time will come very soon."

Ms. Alessandra Z.
Born 1949
Diagnosed with metastases of the liver

She writes in January 1996: "I want you to know that I'm doing well, and that I have no reasons to complain. Many thanks for your tea. Without it, I would no doubt be only a memory."

In April 1996 she adds: "I'm following your diet very scrupulously, and am taking the tea as recommended. I want to live, and I'm willing to sacrifice anything. I'm glad that summer is coming. We have a small garden on the Danube, and my husband has bought some seedlings so I can have all the fresh vegetables I need."

Betty S.
Born 1934
Residence: Chicago, IL.

Diagnosis as of May 23,1996: small lung cancer, stage IV (terminally ill)

She writes to Dr. Reimar C. Breuning on April 21, 1997:

Dear Dr. Bruening,

Because of your great interest and concern in helping hopeless cancer patients I am alive and well today. I will be grateful to you for the rest of my life. Your miraculous herbal tea has made me a miracle statistic. My oncologist cannot believe how a small-cell cancer patient like me, whom he gave three months to live, just celebrated her one-year anniversary looking and feeling so wonderfully healthy, energetic, and happy. And I owe it all to the CoD Tea system, vitamins, and a healthy diet. Before I started taking the tea I was always tired and never wanted to leave the house—quite the opposite of how I had been my entire life. Now I'm a whole human being again, thanks to you.

It will be my pleasure to keep you informed of my well-being. If you have any further questions regarding my medical records please feel free to contact me. I will be happy to assist you in any way possible.

Again, Eternally Grateful,
Betty D.

Afterword

I am pleased to have this opportunity to comment on Dr. Thomas David's research. Before I do, I'd like to address the public's widespread misconception that the practice of phytotherapy (meaning plant medicine; from the Greek *phyton*, plant) and the practice of modern medicine are mutually exclusive. It is unfortunate that such misconceptions are often perceived as truth.

The history of phytotherapy is as old as the history of humans trying to heal themselves. The Sumerians made the earliest sketches on clay tablets depicting the medicinal uses of plants. And the cuneiform writings found in the library of King Assur-banipal depict well over 250 medicinal plants.

Even the Egyptians, whose medical knowledge still astounds us today, were well aware of the healing properties of plants. Then there is the well-known *Ebers Papyrus* which, fifteen hundred years before Christ, collected prescriptions describing over seven hundred plant materials and their uses. The Greeks held plants and their healing properties to be gifts from the gods. And in *The Iliad* Homer told of the well-respected doctors Machaon and Podaleiros, both sons of Asklepios, the god of healing.

Over time the treasury of botanical knowledge faded into obscurity until the eighth century, when the Benedictines gathered together all the existing knowledge of botanical medicine. In her work *Causae et Curae* (causes and cures) the abbess Hildegard von Bingen mentions over sixty-two treatments for fever, seventy-nine for the heart, and ninety-nine for rheumatism and aching joints. But knowledge of the healing powers of plants extended to all levels of society. "Wise women" often possessed an astounding knowledge of the powers of nature. Thousands of them were burned for suspicion of being witches, and as a result much of that knowledge was lost to the world forever. Consequently new plants, substances, and preparations needed to be discovered. Samuel Hahnemann (who developed modern homeopathy), Sebastian Kneipp, and Father Kunzle were important pioneers in this area.

Today, however, phytotherapy has long been considered a science. Modern medicine knows of about three thousand healing plants, about five hundred of which are commonly used for pharmaceutical purposes. Approximately 40 percent of all medications are derived from plant materials or have direct origins to traditional botanical treatments. Scientists have been searching for the mechanisms of these medicinal plants and are working to identify and isolate them. In this respect, recent years have been particularly fruitful. In some cases, we understand more clearly why these plants work the way they do. We must always keep in mind that the whole plant does not necessarily have the same effect as the isolated ingredients. As a rule, the whole plant works less aggressively and more comprehensively than do the isolated active ingredients. Mixing various substances causes them to have varying effects on one another. Depending on the combination, some ingredients may enhance the actions of others, while some may hinder. So we should look at a plant not as a carrier of beneficial substances, but as the beneficial substance itself, the actual healing mechanism. This understanding has been perhaps the greatest advance in recent phytotherapy.

Many plants also display so-called nonspecific, or generic, effects on the human body, as well as on the spirit and soul. These plants stimulate and strengthen the body's natural immune system in ways that we are still trying to understand. It is not yet clear whether such effects are the result of isolated substances or of the synergistic effects of a variety of substances working together.

Nonetheless, plants are not miracle cures. They can only be effective when they are used for their intended purpose, and we must always keep their limitations in mind. Whenever these limitations are either unknown or ignored, modern scientific medicine must step in. The perception of this relationship has led many to believe that there is some kind of competition or animosity between modern medicine and botanical medicine. I hope that a look at the history of botanical medicine and a judicious survey of its present state will reveal that this animosity—with a few exceptions—does not, and should not, exist.

I hope that after the introduction I've just given, you will be surprised to learn that I have followed Dr. David's work from the very beginning. In fourteen years of work, he has been able to define and describe the most important parameters of plant combinations, specifically with regard to their effectiveness, safety, and quality.

These three parameters guarantee safe medical intervention and therapy. I am convinced that Dr. David's preparation provides not just the benefits of individual substances, but the synergistic effects of a combination of natural substances working in concert to strengthen and enhance inherent therapeutic qualities. I do not need to elaborate on the present day importance of strengthening the human immune system. Factors such as environmental pollution, stress, and an unhealthy lifestyle place the immune system under constant attack. In medical treatment, the use of medications having toxic effects on the liver, kidneys, and heart can so weaken the immune system that, in many cases, the negative aspects of treatments such as surgery, chemotherapy, or radiation therapy outweigh any possible benefits, putting the treatments themselves in question, if not suggesting they be ruled out entirely.

Dr. David's system helps to remove toxins from the body, and this in turn leads to a significant strengthening of the immune system. His recommended diet is in itself a huge boost to the body and, in the long term, introduces one potential possibility for the interaction of scientific medicine with natural medicine.

Dr. David's herbal mixture had initial success in animal tests, the promising results of which boded well for its use with humans. Today through word of mouth alone, over two thousand people have been registered and have followed the scientifically based diet and lifestyle changes suggested by Dr. David. On average, most have noticed a marked improvement (weight gain, cessation of pain, lightened spirits, stabilization of condition, partial remission, etc.) within six to eight weeks. Clinically controlled studies with twelve hundred patients have been carried out over two and a half years. The system of conventional methods with concomitant botanical treatment is based upon the most natural of all factors: a healthy, natural, and simply prepared diet, appropriate physical activity, and visualization exercises—all in connection with Dr. David's plant preparation.

From a scientific point of view the synergistic effects of the components of a diverse combination of plants has shown that Dr. David's CoD Tea treatment therapy results in the following four actions: an essential detoxification of the body, a strengthening of the body's immune response, inhibition of tumor growth, and anti-angiogenic effects, which inhibit or halt blood supply to tumors and metastases.

The mechanisms behind the first three of these were easily discerned effects. The fourth function has been identified thanks to the work of Dr. Judah Folkman of Harvard Medical School. Sooner or later he will be honored with a Nobel Prize for his work in the field of anti-angiogenesis.

In conclusion, I am convinced that the holistic botanical system described here—because of its combined effects of encouraging biological immune response, mobilizing the body's natu-ral ability to heal itself, and enhancing the body's own immune system—offers a clear choice for holistic medicine in the fight against the scourge of our overpopulated, poisoned, and immune-weakened society.

Apostolos Georgopoulos, M.D.
Vienna University Clinic of Internal Medicine
Department of Chemotherapy and Experimental and Clinical Microbiology

Postscript

I met Dr. David in January 1995 during a conference on medicinal plant research in San Francisco. At that time I worked as chief scientist with a pharmaceutical company in the Bay Area that specialized in the development of new pharmaceuticals from traditional folk-medicinal sources. He approached me to find out whether my company would be interested in developing his CoD cancer treatment system for the U.S. market. Unfortunately, my company was not pursuing cancer therapy, so I had to decline. Admittedly, I was also quite skeptical after listening to several of his success stories from his efforts in Hungary and Austria; it simply sounded too good to be true! But a strong curiosity remained, and I finally called him up in Vienna and asked for transcripts of his research data, the patient testimonials, and his diet plan. The several pounds of paper that I received a few days later contained information that was not only put together with high integrity, but was nothing short of sensational: here were well-documented cases of patients with stage IV cancer that had become unresponsive to all chemotherapy and radiation treatments, too weak to walk, too sick to eat, with a life prognosis of weeks rather than years, patients that had been sent home to die or who were spending their remaining days immobilized in hospital beds. All of them had begun the CoD system, while their clinical data were strictly monitored, and within weeks their vital signs had begun to improve, increased appetite had resulted in weight gain, and white blood cell counts were significantly increased in several cases. Most importantly, all patients reported a dramatic change in their outlook on life, a replacement of despair and lethargy with optimism, and a will to live.

A month later I left my position and started my own company to introduce plant-based specialties from Europe to the United States, remedies that had proved their efficacy to me over and over in the years when I was still a practicing pharmacist in Munich. I knew that I wanted the CoD system to become part of my product portfolio. Consequently, in July 1995 I traveled to Vienna and met Dr. David and many of his scientific collaborators. I suggested several studies that would prove the stimulating action of CoD upon the immune system and help pinpoint the biomolecular mechanism of action. Moreover, we agreed to begin a pilot study in the U.S., whereby I would offer to patients with advanced cancer free enrollment in a tightly monitored study with the CoD system functioning as a supplement to their present conventional therapies. With the consent of the treating physicians, these patients would take the CoD tea and change their diet according to Dr. David's plan. The tea would be provided free of charge in return for all medical transcripts and testimonials, which the Vienna team would use for their own documentation.

Upon my return I began to recruit candidates through the cancer discussion groups on the Internet, and starting in November 1995, the first patients received the CoD tea. So far I have supported fifteen patients; their diagnoses ranged from small-cell lung carcinoma with liver metastases to cancer of the prostate with metastases in the pelvic bones. I have seen highly metastatic breast cancer and advanced non-Hodgkin's lymphoma. All of these patients had one fact in common: they all were in or close to the terminal stage of their disease; their official prognoses never exceeded a few months. I have collected data and testimonials that are very encouraging for me and completely mirror those that were collected by Dr. David in Europe: in most of these cases the individuals experienced an almost immediate increase in appetite, followed by considerable weight gain and the recovered ability to move around, go to movies, or attend invitations—in other words, a return to a close-to-normal rhythm of life. It was this "improvement of life quality" that convinced me of the merits of Dr. David's approach. Of course, these are very ill people, and in some cases the CoD system came simply too late; it is no surprise that six of my initial group of fifteen have died. However, while still alive all six individuals enjoyed several months of life with a quality that they had not experienced in far too long a time.

I have meanwhile moved from the West Coast to Massachusetts and joined another pharmaceutical company that is exploring the genetics of cancer to identify new pharmaceutical targets. During my research activities here I met Dr. Judah Folkman of Harvard Children's Hospital, a world-renowned authority in the field of angiogenesis, the formation of new blood capillaries. After I described the CoD tea to Dr. Folkman he suggested to test it for anti-angiogenic activity because he suspected that such a mechanism of action might at least be partly responsible for CoD's spectrum of pharmacological effects. I communicated this suggestion to Dr. David and he initiated a corresponding study. The results showed just what Dr. Folkman had suspected: CoD tea inhibits the formation of new blood vessels; as a result, tumors can become starved of oxygen and potential nutrients, resulting in reduced growth or even shrinkage.

All available scientific data point in four directions of CoD action: stimulation of specific white blood cells and the concomitant release of peptides of the interleukin family that directly or indirectly influence tumor growth; stimulation of anti-angiogenic factors (eventually even the same interleukins) that inhibit the formation of nutrient-carrying blood vessels to the tumor masses; the stimulation of endorphins, neuropeptides that modulate pain sensation and are directly or indirectly responsible for the subjective experience of "well being"; and the stimulation of appetite and the suppression of chemotherapy-related nausea, followed by weight gain and improved muscular strength—again, at least partly traceable to the biochemical action of interleukins and endorphins. While these data begin to form a comprehensible pattern, more research must be done until all stones of this intriguing mosaic are in place. Meanwhile, Dr. David's astounding CoD tea will continue to deliver a promise to many more people in desperate need for improvement of their medical situation.

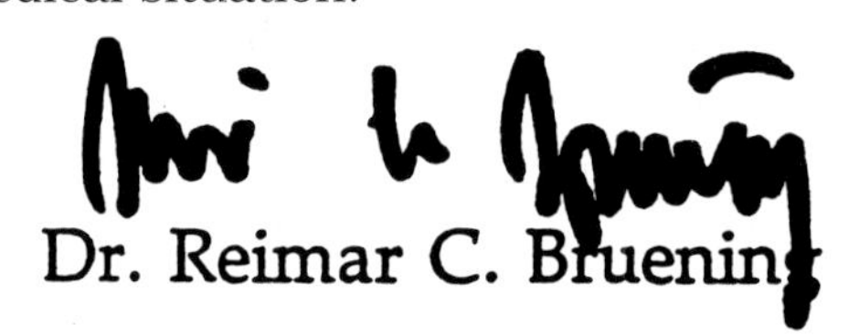

Reimar C. Bruening, Ph.D., R.Ph.
Cambridge, Massachusetts
July 1997

Clinical Evaluation of CoD Tea

Conclusion of clinical testing on the influence of CoD Tea extract on granulocyte function with respect to adherence, chemokinesis, and phagocyte behavior in vivo. The goal of these tests was to test for a putative effect of CoD Tea on lymphocyte functions, adherence, chemokinesis, and phagocyte behavior. Seven subjects took part in the study. Each of the subjects took the prescribed amounts of CoD Tea for a period of fourteen weeks.

Medical background: Blood and other tissues provide an attractive breeding ground for viruses, bacteria, fungi, and parasites. Natural barriers, such as skin and mucous membranes, provide the first level of defense against these microorganisms, insuring that they do not enter the body. There are other defenses in place once some of these germs have penetrated the first line of defense. Together, these defenses are known as the immune system. Antibodies are an effective means of defense against intruders such as virus particles, bacteria, or their toxic byproducts which have penetrated the first line of defense. If these microorganisms actually penetrate on the cellular level, antibodies are no longer of any help. If an intruder has reached this point, there is another line of defense: the macrophages. These so-called "effector cells" can attack foreign microorganisms. This is done with the help of special information cells (T-cells) produced by the macrophages, which contain foreign cells. Along with the destruction of the afflicted host cells by the macrophages, the invading cells and the source of the infection are effectively removed. Until recently we could not influence this immune mechanism, but we have since developed the means for testing both in vivo and in vitro, primarily with granulocytes. This system enables us to observe the activity and migration and phagocytosis of macrophages. In this manner, we can evaluate the effectiveness of various pharmaceuticals as well as, for example, the effects of radicals of the organism.

Results: We attempted to define changes of adherence, motility, and the rate of phagocytosis in nine trials. Levels were measured before and after the application of CoD Tea. In the case of the rate of phagocytosis, levels were measured at three different points: 10, 15, and 20 minutes after incubation.

Effects of CoD Tea as measured by levels of adherence, motility, and rate of phagocytosis.

Patient	Time of measurement	Adherence (%)	Motility* (cm/15 min.)	Phagocytosis (particles/granulocyte) after incubation of: 10 min.	15 min.	20 min.
A	before tea	76.3	7.9	0.84	0.95	1.47
	after tea	80.0	9.0	1.31	2.07	2.64
B	before tea	72.7	12.5	1.26	1.71	2.42
	after tea	85.2	12.1	2.53	2.71	2.98
C	before tea	52.8	7.7	0.92	1.78	2.12
	after tea	88.4	11.4	1.71	2.19	2.35
D	before tea	70.4	11.6	2.36	2.80	3.00
	after tea	89.4	13.8	2.36	2.98	3.10
E	before tea	68.1	8.2	2.35	2.67	3.09
	after tea	87.6	8.4	2.93	3.38	3.54
F	before tea	86.6	11.0	1.00	1.85	1.84
	after tea	91.0	12.5	1.13	2.00	2.51
G	before tea	77.9	11.1	0.92	1.08	1.45
	after tea	92.0	11.3	1.56	1.80	2.28

Adherence: After introduction of CoD Tea granulocyte adherence increased an average of 15.4 percent (ranging from 3.7 to 35.6 percent).

Motility: Change in motility was measured as the change in the distance covered in centimeters per 15-minute increments. This value increased a mean of 1.2 centimeters, with a range of 0.4 to 3.7 centimeters.

Phagocytosis: Phagocytosis was measured as a ratio of particles to granulocytes. Again, after CoD Tea was administered, granulocyte phagocytosis increased in all seven tests. Values were measured at 10, 15, and 20 minutes, and phagocytosis increased in all nine tests. The measured values were nearly double those taken before CoD Tea was administered. At each of the three time points the increase in phagocytosis was 0.6 particles/granulocyte, ranging from 0.13 to 1.37 (10 minutes), 0.18 to 1.12 (15 minutes), and 0.1 to 1.17 (20 minutes) particles to granulocytes.

Conclusion: The results of these tests clearly demonstrate that the application of CoD Tea results in a significant increase in all functions measured. The beneficial in vivo effect on the granulocytes results in an improved immune response. More extensive tests will be needed in order to quantify these effects. In any case, CoD Tea stimulates the immune system of the organism at the cellular level without the side effects of existing synthetic pharmaceuticals. CoD Tea extract appears to have a decidedly positive effect on the organism.

Dr. Peter Schleicher
Medical Chief
Zytognost Munich,
Immunobiology Laboratory
March 1996

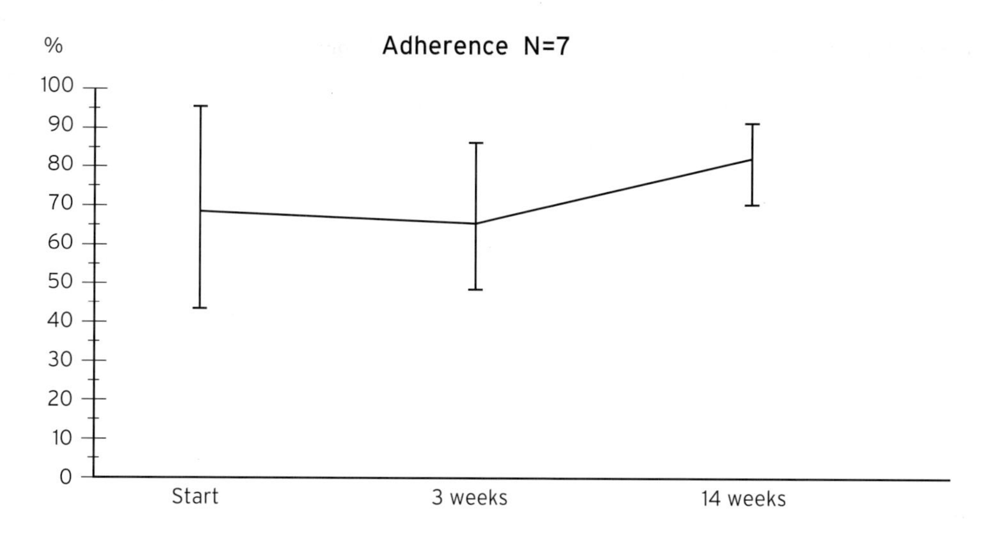

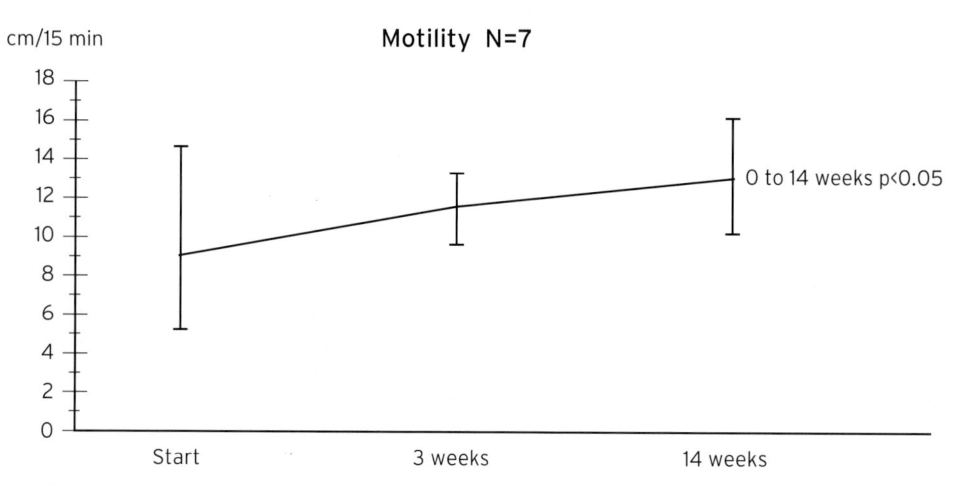

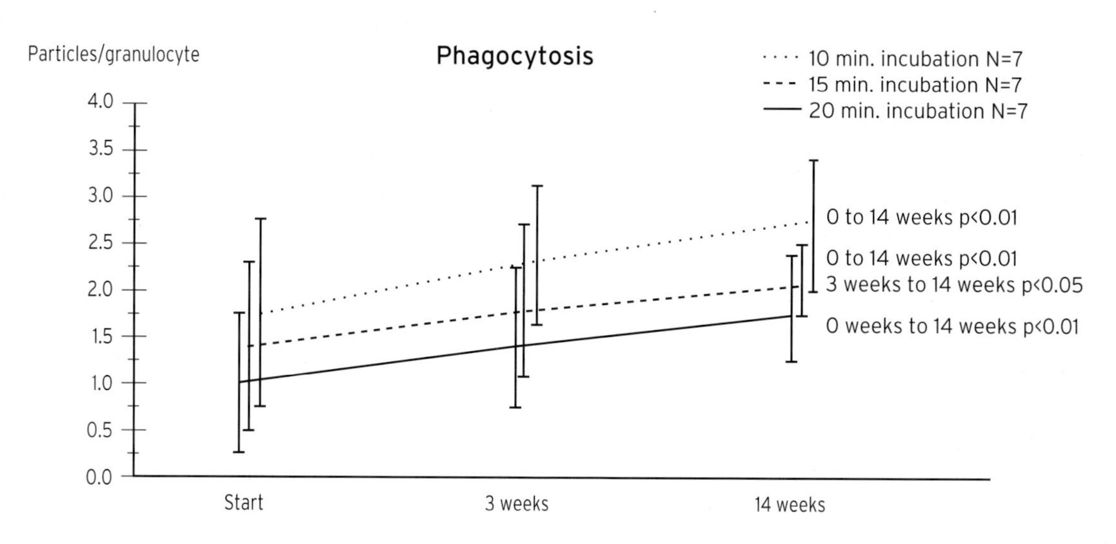

These graphs clearly show the positive effects of CoD Tea on granulocytosis.

Feasibility Study: The Effect of CoD Tea

CELLControl
Biomedical Laboratories, Inc.
June 25, 1997

Dear Dr. David,

Here are the first results of our feasibility study of the CoD Tea on actual cancer cells of a patient.

We received the cancer cells from The Clinic Grosshadern/ Munich to determine chemosensitivity. The patient suffers from metastatic breast cancer, and has already been treated with chemotherapy.

CELLControl performed the Pmc-test on the cancer cells two hours after they had been surgically removed from the patient's spine. This test combines the cancer cells of the patient with a microchip, so that the metabolic activity of the pharmacological effectiveness of different Cytostatica can be measured. In this investigation some very interesting observations were made.

The classic Cytostaticum Epirubicin showed *no effect* on the patient's cells. On the contrary, the cancer cells were resistant to the medication. Indeed, so resistant that the growth of the cancer cells was actually stimulated.

In a control study we tried to determine the effect of CoD Tea on Epirubicin. It was noted that the combination of CoD Tea and Epirubicin showed a resistance dissolving effect. By adding the CoD Tea in a 1:100 ratio, growth stimulation was changed to *extreme growth-inhibition.*

If these exciting findings can be confirmed in controlled follow-up studies—and much points in that direction—then this would mean a major medical breakthrough. It would open up completely new treatment opportunities for those patients who are already resistant to certain chemotherapy drugs.

Ludwig A. Laxhuber, M.D.
Rainer Metzger, M.D.
CELLControl Biomedical
Laboratories, Inc., Munich

Glossary of Medical Terms

adherence: (from Latin *adhaerer,* to stick, adhere) to become bound together, to take root.
adjuvant: (from Latin *adiuvare,* to support, to help) 1. a substance which, when administered (injected) in combination with an antigen, leads to an overall strengthening of the immune response (e.g., to an increased production of antibodies), or changes the manner in which the immune system functions. 2. (pharmaceutical) a medication (substance) which supports or strengthens the effects of another medication.
alkaloid: nitrogen-containing substance produced in plants, many of which have pharmacological effects. Some are extremely poisonous, but can be extremely effective medications when applied appropriately. They can be narcotic (such as opium alkaloid or cocaine), or effective with infectious illness (such as quinine to treat malaria).
angioma: tumor-like growth of new vascular tissue, caused by dilation of the blood vessels.
antibiotic: substance made from microorganisms, or higher plants or animals, which kills or inhibits the growth of microorganisms. Research has discovered several hundred different types, of which only a few are used to treat infectious illnesses.
antibody: body or substance evoked in the organism after the introduction of an antigen. Antibodies react in the body (in vivo) or in the test tube (in vitro) to neutralize antigens, which gives antibodies an important role in the immune system. They are present for the most part in gammaglobulins in the blood serum. Function: antibodies are the immune system's carriers, which work to neutralize foreign and naturally occuring antigens as well as toxins and viruses.
antigen: substance which is treated by a living organism as "foreign." The presence of antigens triggers a predictable, specific immune response, such as the production of antibodies or immune-assisting lymphocytes.
antimycotic: an agent which affects the growth of fungi. Used for skin, mucosal, and systemic mycosis (an infectious condition caused by fungi).
antituberculin: a germ-inhibiting, antibacterial agent used in chemotherapy (a class of acidic, immovable, oxygen-rich, rod-shaped bacteria). There are thirty known types, such as Mycobacterium tuberculosis and Mycobacterium leprae.
astringent: an agent which contracts tissue and controls bleeding and secretion or discharge.
bacterium: any prokaryotic, single-cell life forms with no nuclei, in which genetic material is organized in the form of a pronucleus, which is not separated from the cell plasma by a nuclear membrane. The bacterium are of great importance as assimilators of various metabolic processes, such as fermentation, decay, and illnesses. The eubacteria (true bacteria) are among the smallest life forms. They reproduce by cell division, and can be round, rod-shaped, or spiral.
biochemistry: physiological and biological chemistry; the study of the chemistry of living organs and life processes (such as respiration, metabolism, digestion, excretion, internal and external secretions).
biosynthesis: the formation of various chemical compounds in living cells to facilitate and maintain normal processes and functions of the organism.
carcinogen: substance or agent which, in animal or human tests, increases the incidence of malignant or spontaneously appearing tumors, or which can significantly alter (increase) the range of a tumor in bodily tissue.
carcinogenic: cancer-causing.
carcinoma: malignant tumor originating in the skin.

cardiotoxic: general term for any substance harmful to the heart.
chemotherapeutic agent: general term for naturally occuring or synthetic substances which manifest selectively harmful effects on pathogens and/or tumor cells by blocking metabolism. Types: antibiotics, antimycotics, antituberculins, parasiticides.
chemotherapy: treatment of disease with drugs or chemical substances which inhibit specific pathogens or tumor cells.
coumarin: aromatic substance found in numerous plants, which has anticoagulant, anti-inflammatory, and antiedematous properties.
cystoscopy: examination of the urinary bladder and ureter with a cystoscope, a hollow metal tube which can also take tissue samples (biopsy) and be used for carrying out certain forms of therapy in the bladder (bladder tumors, inflammation).
cytostatic: a group of cytotoxic structures of various chemical origins which inhibit growth and reproduction of active cells.
cytotoxic: damaging to cells.
edema: (Greek for "swelling") painless, noninflammatory swelling due to the accumulation of excess fluid in spaces between tissues, for example in the skin or mucous membranes. Formed by excess hydrostatic pressure from, for example, thrombosis, heart failure, sodium or water retention (common in pregnancy or premenstrually), liver damage, hunger, or damage to capillary walls.
glucocorticoid: one of the three groups of steroid-hormones produced in the adrenal gland. The most important naturally occuring types are: cortisol (hydrocortisone, physiologically the most important of the glucocorticoids), cortisone, and corticosterone. Among the effects are stimulation of glucose production (formation of carbohydrates from amino acids), maintenance of blood sugar levels, and stress reduction.
glycoside: organic compounds containing acetate (similar to ether) from substances in the hydroxyl group. They are classified according to sugar content as glycoside (the most common), galactoside, mannoside, etc.
granulocytes: member of the leukocyte family, multiple-nucleated cell, able to ingest other microorganisms and foreign antigens (and possibly other types of tumor cells and virus-infected cells) by phagocytosis. Granulocytes play a central role in the immune system and are important against infections related to worms and other parasites.
hemangioma: benign blood vessel tumor.
hemoglobin: red blood cells.
hepatotoxic: harmful to the liver.
herpes: (from the Greek for "spreading skin eruption") Any of various skin or mucous conditions. *Herpes simplex:* a harmless, viral skin condition, manifested in clusters of small, needle-sized blisters in the mouth *(H. labialis)* or genitals *(H. progenitalis)*, which clears up a few days after appearing. Herpes simplex virus tends to lie dormant after initial infection, and can become active from such causes as fever (especially resulting from lung or kidney infections or malaria), excessive exposure to the sun, or menstruation.
immune response: general term for the organism's reaction to the presence of a foreign body or substance (antigen). Immune response can include the production of antibodies or immune-assisting lymphocytes.
implantation: 1. introduction or grafting of foreign materials into a body. 2. nidation: embedding a fertilized ovum in the uterus.
in vitro: outside of the organism, in an artificial environment (in a test tube).
in vivo: (from the latin for "in the living") in the body of a living organism.
laser: acronym for *l*ight *a*mplification by *s*timulated *e*mission of *r*adiation; strengthening of light by stimulated emission. A method of creating monochromatic, coherent, nearly parallel light rays with an extremely high energy field. Used in medicine to promote tissue coagulation . The concentrated beam makes lasers especially useful in treating detached retinas, growths in the eye, and growths on the skin.
laser surgery: surgical use of laser to remove tumors in the face and in the larynx. (CO_2 lasers have a remarkable cutting ability and minimize coagulation.) Laser surgery promotes coagulation in tissue with a high percentage of blood vessels up to a depth of approximately 1 millimeter through the transformation of light energy to heat energy.

leukemia: (from Greek *leukos*, white, and *haima*, blood) malignant condition of the white blood cells resulting in excess production of abnormal white blood cells. There are two types in humans: myeloid leukemia, which affects the bone marrow and is marked by a proliferation of granulocytes, and lymphatic leukemia, which results in increased lymphocyte levels (small white blood cells). There are acute and chronic forms.

Acute myeloid leukemia comes on suddenly with high fever, and is distinguished by a high fever due to sepsis. Chronic lymphatic leukemia is relatively benign and can often be present in a patient for over a decade without being fatal. White blood cell count in vascular blood often exceeds normal levels ten- to twentyfold. This condition is often characterized by the presence of lymphoblasts (immature lymphocytes) which are not found in normal blood. Bone marrow tests typically reveal an increase in leukocyte levels. Leukemia is normally accompanied by a reduction in red blood cell count, which causes a pale coloration of the skin. Other symptoms include swollen lymph nodes and an enlarged spleen. Treatments such as pharmaceuticals, radiation therapy, and blood transfusions help to reduce the white blood cell count and can result in long-term improvement, but complete recovery from leukemia is very rare.

leukocytes: white blood cells. There are three types: granulocytes (60–70%), found in the bone marrow; lymphocytes (20–30%) which are produced in the lymph tissue (spleen, lymph nodes); and monocytes (2–6%), the origin of which is not entirely clear.

lymph: fluid consisting of plasma and free cells, which is introduced to the bloodstream through the lymph vessels. Promotes exchange of oxygen between blood and cells which cannot be reached directly via the capillaries. In tissue it stores metabolic products of cells, and promotes the removal of toxins and foreign bodies to prevent them from entering the bloodstream.

lymph nodes: (formerly incorrectly known as the lymph glands) connected to the lymph system, these tiny, round secondary organs of the lymph system are the most important producers of lymphocytes in adults.

lymph system: a part of the circulatory system, which allows lymph to enter into the bloodstream. In humans and other mammals the lymph system includes the lymph vessels and the lymph nodes.

macrophages: tissue cells, able to eliminate larger particles (bacteria, microorganisms, foreign cells) through phagocytosis.

metabolites: any substance used in metabolism; a substance synthesized in the organism, such as hormones or enzymes.

metastases: (from Greek for "change," "metamorphosis") a second-generation growth accompanying malignant primary growths in the advanced stages of development, often distant from the primary growth. These cells can be transported through the body in the bloodstream, the lymph system, or other channels or orifices, and transported with fluids to a fertile breeding ground (often at first the lungs, and later in bone marrow, liver, brain, skin, or internal organs) to promote the growth of metastases. Metastases can be larger and can cause more serious problems than the primary tumor. The unleashing of a malignant growth accompanied by the release of thousands of tiny second-generation growths follows the breakdown of the immune system. Metastasization refers to the presence of a new location of the disease. Depending on the location of the metastases with respect to the original tumor, they can be characterized as local, regional, or distant.

microbiology: branch of science concerned with microorganisms, their influence on life forms and potential therapies.

microorganism: microbes, small organisms, bacteria, viruses, fungi.

microphages: granulocytes.

migration: 1. movement of cells and foreign bodies within the organism, for example, the movement of neuroblasts (immature nerve cells) from their embryos to a final location in the brain, or leukocytes through the blood vessel walls, or sperm within the cervix. 2. sociology: movement of individuals or groups (immigration, emigration).

monocytes: mononuclear blood cells belonging to the group of leukocytes.

morphine: alkaloid form of opium; a narcotic pain killer.
motility: ability to move.
nephrotoxic: toxic to the kidneys.
parameter: an arbitrary numerical constant used to allow for the practical measurement of outcomes.
parenchyme: essential or functional cells of an organ which allow that organ to carry out its functions.
pericardium: protective covering of the heart, consisting of two layers. Protects against overextension of the heart muscles and the spread of infection.
phagocytes: specialized cells found in the tissue of multicelled animals. Phagocytes have the ability to ingest and neutralize harmful substances (phagocytosis). Depending on the location in the organism and their specialized function, they are called amoebocytes, histiocytes, monocytes, macrophages, fibrocytes, osteoclasts, and chondroclasts.
phagocytosis: engulfing and breaking down (through enzyme action or oxidation) of a foreign cell or microorganism by phagocytes.
pharmaceutical: drug or medication.
pharmacology: the science of the interaction of pharmaceuticals and organisms.
phytotherapy: treatment using plants, plant cells, and plant-derived preparations to treat or prevent illness. Plant medicines have a broad spectrum of action and more mild side effects than synthetic medications.
plasma: living substance (protoplasma). In physiology, a clotting substance, such as blood plasma.
polymorphic nucleus: a cell, such as a leukocyte, with multiple nuclei.
proband: participant in clinical tests examining the efficacy or side effects of medications.
radical: a group of stable atoms with a specific structure in a molecule.
radium therapy: seldom-used form of radiation therapy with Radium 226. Radium "needles" are brought into direct contact with tumor tissue (primarily gynecological tumors).
regression: 1. diminishing of a tumor as a result of therapy. 2. (psychoanalysis) defense mechanism which is manifested in psychological behavior characteristic of childhood or some earlier developmental stage as a reaction to a painful or unbearable situation (for example, with neurosis, schizophrenia, or psychosis).
remission: cessation of symptoms of an illness. A complete or full remission signifies a condition in which therapeutic interventions have succeeded to the point that a positive diagnosis of the disease is no longer possible, and the patient feels totally healthy. A partial remission is characterized by a marked improvement in test results and an overall improvement in condition, but without total normalization of the patient's condition.
synergy: the coordinated interaction of two or more elements (for example, muscles and glands).
synthesis: formation of a new substance or entity from previously existing ones.
thrombocytes: blood platelets; thin, colorless disks approximately .003 millimeter thick. Normal blood contains a concentration of approximately 300,000 to 700,000 per 1 cubic millimeter. Especially important for coagulation (clotting of blood).
toxic: poisonous.
toxins: immunogenic, water-soluble substances which have a variety of harmful effects on microorganisms, plants, and animals.
transplantation: introduction of cells, tissue, or organs from one individual to another, or from one site in one individual to another site in the same individual, i.e. blood transfusion or transplant of cornea, vessels, skin, kidneys, liver, bone marrow, heart, lungs, or other internal organs.
viruses: term for biological structures which are pathogenic (disease-causing) in humans, plants, animals, and bacteria. Viruses share the following characteristics: 1. they contain genetic information in only one form of nucleic acid, either RNA or DNA. 2. they are the smallest, simplest, self-reproducing organisms in nature. They use living cells as host organisms, and infect their hosts with illnesses and disease.

Acknowledgments

I'd like to thank everyone who has helped us with our research in the Amazon and elsewhere. Your assistance—even in our most difficult hours—with heart, deed, and soul has shown us the true meaning of the word friendship. With idealism, unwavering determination, and action you have allowed our small but international group to carry out our work for the betterment of humanity. I extend my most heartfelt thanks to you all.

Abraham, Ilona, Dr.; Arndt, Jürgen, Dr.; Balaun, Ernest, Magg., DDr.; Bathory, Gyoergy, Dr.; Baumgartner, Gerhard, Prim. Doz., Dr.; Bobek, Ernst, Sektionschef, Dr.; Bodrogi, Gyula; Braunschweiger, Jürgen, Dir.; Brazda-Uiterwiyk, Eva, Mag.; Brzica, Halina; Bruening, Reimar C., Dr.; Busek, Erhard, BM a.D.Dr.; Cordes, Susanne, DI; Cserna, Hildegard; Dalheimer, Veronika, Dr.; Diwald, Erhard; deSoglio, Mario; Dohr, Hans-Peter, Mag.; Elhenitzky, Richard, Dr.; Elkan-Stallmeier, Inge; Farkas, Ilona, Dr.; Ferreira, Cid, Dr.; Galfi, Peter, Univ.Prof.Dr.; Gehl, Heinz, Vorstandsdirektor; Georgopoulos, Apostolos, Univ.Prof.DDr.; Geresdorfer, Franz, Regierungsrat; Godoy Perez, Edwin; Graf, Ferdinand, Dr.; Graft, Ernst, KR; Greger, Harald, Univ.Prof.Dr.; Guarniero, Roberto, Prof.Dr.; Gyulavari, Oliver, Dr.; Haider, Ulla, General Secretary; Harant, Ingrid, Dipl.-Tzt.; Harant, Ilse; Häupl, Armin, DI; Hayde, Dieter, DArch; Herrmann, Norbert; Hock, Johannes jun., Dr.; Hofer, Otmar, Univ.Prof.Dr.; Homolya, Laszlo, Dr.; Jäger, Franz Josef, Präsident Dr.; Jandl, Brigitte, Mag.; Jensch, Alexander, Min.Rat.Dr.; Juhasz, Csaba, Dr.; Juhasz, Tamas, Dr.; Kaiser, Katalin, Dr.; Karsai, Ferenc, Prof.Dr.; Kern, Renald, Mag.; Kery, Agnes, Dr.; Keve, Tibor, Dr.; Kohl, Heribert, Dr.; Königshofer, Wolfgang, DDr.; Kovacs, Judit, General Manager; Krischke, Eleonore, Dr.; Kugler, Christian; Kunze, Peter; Kutas, Ferenc, Prof.Dr.; Lage, Lafayette, Doz.Dr.; Leibetseder, Josef, Prof.Dr.; Li, Qin, DDr.; Liebeswar, Gunther, Doz.Dr.; Lischka, Lutz; Loube, Lucie, Präsidentin; Machacek, Rudolf, Dr.; Mangal, Janice; Markus, Georg; Mayer, Alois, Dr.; Mendez Nkuka, Cosmo; Meruk, Jozsef; Mickschе, Michael, Univ.Prof.Dr.; Mock, Alois, BM a.D.Dr.; Mohr, Thomas, Dr.; Neogrady, Zsuzsa, Univ.Doz.Dr.; Osterbauer, Gabriele; Ott, Istvan, Dr.; Padilha Filho, Joao, Prof.Dr.; Parag, Gyula, DI; Pethes, Gyoergy, Prof.Dr.; Pfanhauser, Elfride; Poppe, Hubert; Primus, Alton; Rabl, Peter; Rau, Thomas, Dr.; Reichhart, Freddy; Rozsenich, Norbert, Sektionschef Dr.; Sarkadi, Balazs, Dr.; Schleicher, Peter, Dr.; Schmalhart, Angelika; Schönborn, Benedikt; Schuller, Gerhard, Direktor; Schwarz, Hans, Dr.; Schweiger, Oliver M.; Seisenbacher, Peter; Sellitsch, Siegfried, Dkfm.Dr.; Skotton, Franz Fosef, BR Prof.Dr.; Smetana, Walter, Dr.; Spängler, Peter, Prof.Dr.; Stacher, Alois, Prof.Dr.; Steinitz, Erich, Dr.; Sternberger, Heinrich, Prof.Dr.; Stiegnitz, Peter, Min.Rat.Prof.Dr.; Stöhr, Johannes, Dr.; Stöhr, Rudolf, Dr.; Szabo, Eva, G.; Szendrei, Timea; Szepesi, Kalman, Prof.Dr.; Teicht, Gustav, Dr.; Tesar, Helmuth, Dr.; Tröstl, Heinz, Ing.; Tsur, Itamar, Prof.Dr.; Turi, Ernö, Prof.Dr.; Tusor, Erzsebet, Dr.; Uyka, Dieter, Prof.DI; von Medveczky, Marianne; Varady, Tamas, Dr.; Voith, Ägi; Wagner, Felix, OMR Dr.; Winkler, Brigitte R.; Wodnianski, Peter, Prof.Dr.; Wokurek, Hanns-P., Direktor; Wrbka, Heinrich, Dr.; Zouein, Elias Jean.

Illustration credits

The color photographs were taken by Dr. Thomas David in the rainforests of South America and China. Botanical drawings have been loaned to the author thanks to: Zoran Mujbegovic (pp. 23, 25, 66, 67 (left and center), 68 (center and right), 69, 70, 71, 72); Micha Dragutinovic (pp. 67 (right), 68 (left) 73, 74, 75, 76, 77, 78, 79); Author's archive (pp. 17, 19, 30, 31, 38, 42, 50, 51, 54, 55, 56, 57, 81, 83, 87, 89, 90, 91, 93, 100, 116, 117, 118, 135); Hans D. Dossenbach (p. 8, lower left); Werner Stanzl (p. 120); Archive of the Vienna Standard (p. 108); and Luzerne Central Library (pp. 21, 22, 24, 26, 27, 28, 37, 39, 52).

For more information on the CoD Therapeutic System:

Institute for Immunostabilization Research and Information
c/o MDA, Inc.
150 Fifth Avenue #835
New York, NY 10011
Phone: 212-727-0407
Fax: 212-727-0409
E-mail: codplus@aol.com
Contacts: Baerbel Dainard, Michael Dainard

Or:

Institut zur Immunstabilisierungs-Forschung und Information
Margaretenstrasse 8
A-1040 Wien
Austria
Phone: 43-1-585-18-05
Fax: 43-1-585-18-05-13

For those who would like to discuss the CoD Therapeutic System with a patient who has used it, Ms. Betty Swanson has generously offered her time. She may be contacted in Florida at: 954-425-0138.

Attention: The authors hereby declare that none of the scientific studies described in this book regarding use and effects of the CoDPlus and nutrition system were conducted under supervision of or in any way monitored by the United States Food and Drug Administration (FDA). None of the testimonials published herein were independently verified by FDA-affiliated researchers. The authors do not make any claims regarding the efficacy of CoD in the treatment of any medical condition. The authors do not regard CoD to be a medicine or a therapeutic agent, according to the definitions outlined by the FDA, but part of a dietary regime as a dietary supplement according to the definitions given in the Dietary Supplement Health and Education Act of 1996. Persons who want to partake in this dietary regime are strongly encouraged to discuss this with their treating physicians.